T0176291

Stroke

Stroke

EDITED BY

Kevin M. Barrett, MD, MSc
Mayo Clinic
Jacksonville
FL, USA

James F. Meschia, MD
Mayo Clinic
Jacksonville
FL, USA

NEUROLOGY IN PRACTICE:

SERIES EDITORS: ROBERT A. GROSS, DEPARTMENT OF NEUROLOGY, UNIVERSITY OF ROCHESTER MEDICAL CENTER, ROCHESTER, NY, USA

JONATHAN W. MINK, DEPARTMENT OF NEUROLOGY, UNIVERSITY OF ROCHESTER MEDICAL CENTER, ROCHESTER, NY, USA

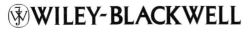

A John Wiley & Sons, Ltd., Publication

This edition first published 2013 © 2013 by John Wiley & Sons

Wiley-Blackwell is an imprint of John Wiley & Sons, formed by the merger of Wiley's global Scientific, Technical and Medical business with Blackwell Publishing.

Registered Office
John Wiley & Sons, Ltd, The Atrium, Southern Gate, Chichester, West Sussex, PO19 8SQ, UK

Editorial Offices
9600 Garsington Road, Oxford, OX4 2DQ, UK
The Atrium, Southern Gate, Chichester, West Sussex, PO19 8SQ, UK
111 River Street, Hoboken, NJ 07030-5774, USA

For details of our global editorial offices, for customer services and for information about how to apply for permission to reuse the copyright material in this book please see our website at www.wiley.com/wiley-blackwell

The right of the author to be identified as the author of this work has been asserted in accordance with the UK Copyright, Designs and Patents Act 1988.

All rights reserved. No part of this publication may be reproduced, stored in a retrieval system, or transmitted, in any form or by any means, electronic, mechanical, photocopying, recording or otherwise, except as permitted by the UK Copyright, Designs and Patents Act 1988, without the prior permission of the publisher.

Designations used by companies to distinguish their products are often claimed as trademarks. All brand names and product names used in this book are trade names, service marks, trademarks or registered trademarks of their respective owners. The publisher is not associated with any product or vendor mentioned in this book. This publication is designed to provide accurate and authoritative information in regard to the subject matter covered. It is sold on the understanding that the publisher is not engaged in rendering professional services. If professional advice or other expert assistance is required, the services of a competent professional should be sought.

The contents of this work are intended to further general scientific research, understanding, and discussion only and are not intended and should not be relied upon as recommending or promoting a specific method, diagnosis, or treatment by physicians for any particular patient. The publisher and the author make no representations or warranties with respect to the accuracy or completeness of the contents of this work and specifically disclaim all warranties, including without limitation any implied warranties of fitness for a particular purpose. In view of ongoing research, equipment modifications, changes in governmental regulations, and the constant flow of information relating to the use of medicines, equipment, and devices, the reader is urged to review and evaluate the information provided in the package insert or instructions for each medicine, equipment, or device for, among other things, any changes in the instructions or indication of usage and for added warnings and precautions. Readers should consult with a specialist where appropriate. The fact that an organization or Website is referred to in this work as a citation and/or a potential source of further information does not mean that the author or the publisher endorses the information the organization or Website may provide or recommendations it may make. Further, readers should be aware that Internet Websites listed in this work may have changed or disappeared between when this work was written and when it is read. No warranty may be created or extended by any promotional statements for this work. Neither the publisher nor the author shall be liable for any damages arising herefrom.

Library of Congress Cataloging-in-Publication Data
Stroke / edited by Kevin M. Barrett, James F. Meschia.
    p. ; cm. – (Neurology in practice)
  Includes bibliographical references and index.
  ISBN 978-0-470-67436-9 (pbk. : alk. paper)
I. Barrett, Kevin M.   II. Meschia, James F.   III. Series: Neurology in practice.
[DNLM: 1. Stroke–diagnosis.   2. Stroke–therapy.   3. Acute Disease.
4. Secondary Prevention.   WL 356]
  616.8′1-dc23
                                 2012044839
A catalogue record for this book is available from the British Library.

Wiley also publishes its books in a variety of electronic formats. Some content that appears in print may not be available in electronic books.

Cover image: Main image: © http://iStockphoto.com/Eraxion; inset Fig. 5.1 with kind permission from Andreas H. Kramer
Cover design by Sarah Dickinson

Set in 8.75/11.75pt Utopia by SPi Publisher Services, Pondicherry, India
Printed and bound in Malaysia by Vivar Printing Sdn Bhd

1   2013

Contents

Color plates are found facing page 22

Contributors

Nader Antonios, MBChB, MPH&TM
Assistant Professor
Department of Neurology
College of Medicine-Jacksonville
University of Florida
Jacksonville
FL, USA

Karthik Arcot, MD
Neuro-Interventional Fellow
Lutheran Medical Center
Brooklyn
NY, USA

Kevin M. Barrett, MD, MSc
Assistant Professor of Neurology
Department of Neurology
Mayo Clinic
Jacksonville
FL, USA

Samir R. Belagaje, MD
Assistant Professor
Departments of Neurology and
Rehabilitation Medicine
Emory University School of Medicine
Atlanta
GA, USA

Andrew J. Butler, PT, MBA, PhD, FAHA
Associate Dean of Research and Professor
B.F. Lewis School of Nursing and Health
Professions
Georgia State University
Atlanta
GA, USA

Bart M. Demaerschalk, MD, MSc, FRCP(C)
Professor of Neurology
Director, Cerebrovascular Diseases Center
Director, Teleneurology and Telestroke Program
Divisions of Vascular, Hospital, and Critical Care
Neurology
Department of Neurology
Mayo Clinic
Phoenix
AZ, USA

Bryan J. Eckerle, MD
Department of Neurology
University of Virginia Health System
Charlottesville
VA, USA

Kelly Flemming, MD
Mayo Clinic College of Medicine
Rochester
MN, USA

Jason M. Johnson, MD
Diagnostic Neuroradiology Clinical Fellow
Massachusetts General Hospital/
Harvard Medical School
Boston
MA, USA

Andreas H. Kramer, MD, MSc, FRCPC
Clinical Assistant Professor
Departments of Critical Care Medicine and Clinical
Neurosciences
Hotchkiss Brain Institute, Foothills Medical Center
University of Calgary
Calgary
AB, Canada

Michael H. Lev, MD
Associate Radiologist, Diagnostic Neuroradiology
Associate Professor of Radiology,
Harvard Medical School
Massachusetts General Hospital
Boston
MA, USA

James F. Meschia, MD
Professor and Chair
Department of Neurology
Mayo Clinic Florida
Jacksonville
FL, USA

Raid G. Ossi, MD
Research Fellow
Department of Neurology
Mayo Clinic
Jacksonville
FL, USA

Scott Silliman, MD
Associate Professor
Department of Neurology
College of Medicine-Jacksonville
University of Florida
Jacksonville
FL, USA

Andrew M. Southerland, MD, MSc
Department of Neurology
University of Virginia Health System
Charlottesville
VA, USA

Albert J. Yoo, MD
Assistant Radiologist, Diagnostic and
Interventional Neuroradiology
Assistant Professor of Radiology
Harvard Medical School
Massachusetts General Hospital
Boston
MA, USA

Series Foreword

The genesis for this book series started with the proposition that, increasingly, physicians want direct, useful information to help them in clinical care. Textbooks, while comprehensive, are useful primarily as detailed reference works but pose challenges for uses at the point of care. By contrast, more outline-type references often leave out the "hows and whys" – pathophysiology, pharmacology – that form the basis of management decisions. Our goal for this series is to present books, covering most areas of neurology, that provide enough background information to allow the reader to feel comfortable, but not so much as to be overwhelming; and to associate that with practical advice from experts about care, combining the growing evidence base with best practices.

Our series will encompass various aspects of neurology, with topics and the specific content chosen to be accessible and useful.

Chapters cover critical information that will inform the reader of the disease processes and mechanisms as a prelude to treatment planning. Algorithms and guidelines are presented, when appropriate. "Tips and Tricks" boxes provide expert suggestions, while other boxes present cautions and warnings to avoid pitfalls. Finally, we provide "Science Revisited" sections that review the most important and relevant science background material, and "Bibliography" sections that guide the reader to additional material.

We welcome feedback. As additional volumes are added to the series, we hope to refine the content and format so that our readers will be best served.

Our thanks, appreciation, and respect go out to our editors and their contributors, who conceived and refined the content for each volume, assuring a high-quality, practical approach to neurological conditions and their treatment.

Our thanks also go to our mentors and students (past, present, and future), who have challenged and delighted us; to our book editors and their contributors, who were willing to take on additional work for an educational goal; and to our publisher, Martin Sugden, for his ideas and support for wonderful discussions and commiseration over baseball and soccer teams that might not quite have lived up to expectations. We would like to dedicate the series to Marsha, Jake, and Dan; and to Janet, Laura, and David. And also to Steven R. Schwid, MD, our friend and colleague, whose ideas helped to shape this project and whose humor brightened our lives, but he could not complete this goal with us.

Robert A. Gross
Jonathan W. Mink
Rochester, July 2011

Preface

Stroke is a medical emergency. Rapid bedside diagnosis and interpretation of neuroimaging studies is necessary to identify patients eligible for acute stroke therapies. Identification of the stroke mechanism in conjunction with prompt initiation of appropriate preventative strategies reduces the risk of recurrence. The acute stroke care continuum typically concludes with early establishment of rehabilitation and recovery programs. The purpose of this book is to give providers an evidence-based roadmap that they can use at the bedside for the care of patients with acute stroke.

Each chapter is authored by physicians with experience and expertise in the front-line evaluation and treatment of patients affected by stroke. The content of each chapter is comprehensive, but not exhaustive, which facilitates utility as both a reference and point-of-care resource. Key references have been included, but limited in number, so as to not interfere with readability. Content included in "Tips and Tricks" and "Science Revisited" boxes direct the reader to clinical pearls and the scientific basis supporting key recommendations. An appendix is included for easy access to validated prognostic scales and measures of stroke severity and disability.

We wish to thank Drs. Gross and Mink for the opportunity to edit this book and the staff at Wiley-Blackwell publishing for guiding us through the process of crafting the content outline, inviting expert authors, and final editing. Without their vision and encouragement a project of this magnitude would not have been possible.

We dedicate this book to stroke patients, their families, and their care givers – past, present, and future.

Kevin M. Barrett
James F. Meschia

Bedside Evaluation of the Acute Stroke Patient

Bryan J. Eckerle, MD and Andrew M. Southerland, MD, MSc

Department of Neurology, University of Virginia Health System, Charlottesville, Virginia

Introduction

Emanating from the results of the original National Institute of Neurological Disorders and Stroke recombinant tissue plasminogen activator (NINDS rt-PA) trial [1], the management of acute stroke has evolved as a cornerstone of emergency medical care, hospital medicine, and clinical neurology. While the only treatment for acute ischemic stroke approved by the US Food and Drug Administration (FDA) remains intravenous (IV) rt-PA administered within 3 hours of symptom onset, the field continues to expand with a focus on more timely treatment, expanding the pool of patients eligible for treatment, and optimization of methods of reperfusion. These advances include the use of IV rt-PA beyond the 3-hour window, the direct administration of intra-arterial rt-PA, and implementation of a variety of devices aimed at mechanical thrombectomy and other interventional means of cerebrovascular recanalization. However, integrating all of the scientific evidence guiding the acute stroke paradigm is daunting, even for the most seasoned vascular neurologist. According to the National Guideline Clearinghouse, an initiative of the Agency for Healthcare Research and Quality in the Department of Health and Human Services, there are currently 225 published guidelines related to "acute stroke" from various organizations and societies around the world [2]. The current standard of stroke care in the US is guided by the American Heart Association/American Stroke Association's (AHA/ASA) Get With the Guidelines (GWTG) program [3].

While stroke therapeutics will be discussed in detail elsewhere in this book, the aim of this chapter is to offer a simple, practical approach to the bedside evaluation of the acute stroke patient. As the opinions and recommendations herein draw on experience treating acute stroke, they also reflect the literature and guiding evidence. The chapter will broadly highlight seminal studies, published AHA/ASA guidelines, FDA regulations, and The Joint Commission (TJC) certification requirements for primary/comprehensive stroke centers – links to further resources can be found in the Appendix, Chapter 9. Explored in detail will be the various issues facing neurologists or other physicians in acute stroke scenarios, including an accurate gathering of history, essentials of the acute stroke physical exam, radiological diagnosis, and potential hurdles precluding a treatment decision. While these necessary steps are very much protocol driven, the reality of the acute stroke setting dictates a somewhat simultaneous process in order to achieve the efficient delivery of treatment. Ultimately, the aim of the chapter is to further promote rapid diagnosis and timely management for all acute stroke patients, as the medical community continues to strive for the best possible outcomes from this disabling and deadly disease.

Is it a stroke?

Despite rapid advances in neuroimaging over the past 20 years, the bedrock of the evaluation of the acute stroke patient remains sound clinical diagnosis. The physician is frequently asked to see a

Stroke, First Edition. Edited by Kevin M. Barrett and James F. Meschia.
© 2013 John Wiley & Sons, Ltd. Published 2013 by John Wiley & Sons, Ltd.

patient in urgent consultation for treatment of acute stroke in the absence of a firmly established diagnosis. Even with the advent of highly advanced neuroimaging techniques, *stroke* remains a clinical diagnosis; as opposed to an *infarct*, which is an imaging or tissue-based diagnosis. Stroke is, by definition, the acute onset of a persistent focal neurological deficit or constellation of deficits referable to a specific cerebrovascular territory. The absence of abrupt onset of symptoms all but precludes acute stroke as the diagnosis. Symptoms that do not all fit into a specific vascular territory suggest either a diagnosis other than stroke or the possibility of multifocal ischemia as may be seen in cardioembolism. Additionally, stroke typically produces *negative* symptoms –that is to say, loss of strength, sensation, vision, or other neurological function. Presence of *positive* symptoms (paresthesias, involuntary movements, visual phenomena) is uncommon in stroke, unless the patient with a cortical stroke is having a concurrent seizure or occasionally a triggered migraine – as in cervical artery dissection.

Ischemic stroke subtypes in specific vascular territories tend to produce fairly predictable constellations of signs and symptoms, or "syndromes" [4]. Rapid recognition of these syndromes is crucial in early diagnosis and timely treatment of acute stroke or, often of equal importance, the elimination of stroke as a potential diagnosis. In terms of broadly defined clinical stroke syndromes, one can consider large vessel versus small vessel presentations. Generally speaking, large vessel strokes tend to occur in the setting of atherosclerotic and/or embolic disease, whereas small vessel (lacunar) strokes tend to present in the setting of chronic small vessel occlusive disease related primarily to chronic hypertension and diabetes. The clinical manifestations of commonly encountered large vessel syndromes are described in Table 1.1.

Table 1.1 Large vessel stroke syndromes (laterality assumes left hemispheric dominance)

Vascular territory	Signs and symptoms
Internal carotid artery (ICA)	Combined ACA/MCA syndromes; ipsilateral monocular visual loss secondary to central retinal artery occlusion (amaurosis); branch retinal artery occlusions may present as ipsilesional altitudinal field cuts
Left anterior cerebral artery (ACA)	Right leg numbness and weakness, transcortical motor aphasia, and possibly ipsilesional or contralesional ideomotor apraxia
Right ACA	Left leg numbness and weakness, motor neglect, and possibly ipsilesional or contralesional ideomotor apraxia
Left middle cerebral artery (MCA)	Right face/arm > leg numbness and weakness, aphasia, left gaze preference
Right MCA	Left face/arm > leg numbness and weakness, left hemispatial neglect, right gaze preference, agraphesthesia, stereoagnosia
Left posterior cerebral artery (PCA)	Complete or partial right homonymous hemianopsia, alexia without agraphia; if midbrain involvement, ipsilateral 3rd nerve palsy with mydriasis and contralateral hemiparesis (Weber syndrome)
Right PCA	Complete or partial left homonymous hemianopsia (same as above if midbrain involvement)
Superior cerebellar artery (SCA)	Ipsilesional limb and gait ataxia
Anterior inferior cerebellar artery (AICA)	Vertigo and ipsilesional deafness, possibly also ipsilesional facial weakness and ataxia
Vertebral/posterior inferior cerebellar artery (PICA)	Ipsilesional limb and gait ataxia; if lateral medullary involvement can have Wallenberg syndrome (see Table 1.4)
Basilar artery (BA)	Pontine localization with impaired lateral gaze, horizontal diplopia and dysconjugate gaze, nonlocalized hemiparesis, dysarthria

The syndromes above reflect classical neuroanatomy and may vary depending on individual variations in the circle of Willis or collateral vascular supply.

Cortical syndromes

Between large vessel and cardioembolic disease, there are several classic cortical syndromes that when presenting acutely are most often the result of an ischemic stroke. The classic hallmark of a left hemispheric cortical syndrome involves aphasia. Aphasia is defined as an acquired abnormality of *language* in any form. By and large, aphasia presents as a deficit of verbal language, but truly involves any medium of communication (e.g. reading and writing, or sign language in the hearing impaired). Specific linguistic properties that may be affected by aphasia include volume of speech, vocabulary, cadence, syntax, and phonics. Often, subtle aphasia is difficult to distinguish from encephalopathy and it is important for the bedside clinician to test specific domains of language – fluency, repetition, comprehension, naming, reading, and writing – in order to make the correct diagnosis.

Specific types of aphasia most often encountered in stroke patients (Table 1.2) classically include expressive/motor/nonfluent (Broca's) and receptive/ sensory/fluent (Wernicke's) types. Strokes causing expressive aphasia localize to the posterior inferior frontal lobe, or frontal operculum, whereas receptive aphasias commonly originate from lesions in the posterior superior temporal/inferior parietal lobe. Both of these types commonly affect naming and repetition. Broca's patients are best identified by difficulties with word finding, speech initiation, volume of speech, and in making paraphasic errors (e.g. "hassock" instead of "hammock"). Wernicke's patients have clearly impaired comprehension with nonsensical speech, but preserved speech volume and cadence. The transcortical aphasias mirror motor and sensory types except in preservation of repetition, due to lack of injury to the arcuate fasciculus linking Broca's and Wernicke's areas.

Figure 1.1 displays the "aphasia box" showing the overlap between the commonly encountered aphasias.

> ★ TIPS AND TRICKS
>
> A common false localizer for aphasia is left thalamic stroke, which may present with a mixed aphasia of nonspecific character.

In the bedside evaluation of the stroke patient, differentiating between aphasia subtypes is less relevant than differentiating aphasia from encephalopathy. As most all aphasia emanates from dominant hemispheric injury, commonly middle cerebral artery (MCA) occlusion, one should consider the abrupt onset of aphasia indicative of stroke until proven otherwise.

> ★ TIPS AND TRICKS
>
> Aphasia differs from delirium (acute confusional state) in that attention is usually preserved in isolated aphasia. Moreover, the aphasic patient is often visibly aware of and frustrated by their deficits, as opposed to the poorly attentive patient with encephalopathy.

If aphasia is the hallmark of dominant (*left*) hemisphere cortical injury, then hemispatial neglect is the hallmark of injury in the nondominant (*right*) hemisphere. Accordingly, abrupt onset of hemineglect should raise concern for acute stroke by occlusion of the right MCA. Examining the patient with neglect at the bedside is challenging, primarily due to difficulties in teasing out primary contralateral motor weakness and numbness. The most sensitive bedside test for subtle neglect is

Table 1.2 The aphasias

	Fluency	Comprehension	Repetition
Motor/expressive (Broca)	Impaired	Normal	Impaired
Sensory/receptive (Wernicke)	Normal	Impaired	Impaired
Conduction	Normal	Normal	Impaired
Transcortical motor	Impaired	Normal	Normal
Transcortical sensory	Normal	Impaired	Normal
Mixed	Variable	Variable	Variable
Global	Impaired	Impaired	Impaired

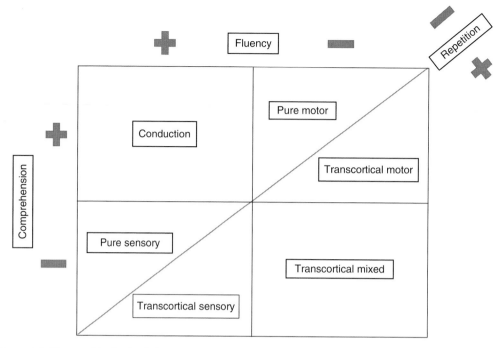

Figure 1.1 The graphical aphasia box.

double simultaneous stimulation to look for *extinction* of contralateral sensory modalities. In other words, when presented with bilateral stimuli, the neglectful patient will preferentially identify the ipsilateral stimulus, often in the absence of a primary sensory deficit (see National Institutes of Health Stroke Scale (NIHSS) item 11, in the Appendix, Chapter 9). Extinction may include not only tactile sensation but also other sensory modalities, such as vision or hearing. Motor neglect is typified by preferential use of the ipsilateral limbs when formal confrontational testing reveals no actual hemiparesis. The tactful bedside clinician, when asking the patient to raise both limbs, may observe a delay in or absence of activation of the contralateral side.

Making the evaluation of the neglectful patient more difficult still is the frequent accompaniment of agnosia. These patients may lack awareness of their deficit (*anosagnosia*) and may seem apathetic to the gravity of their situation. Other nondominant hemispheric phenomena may include stereoagnosia (inability to identify an object by touch), agraphesthesia (deficit of dermal kinesthesia tested by tracing numbers or letters on the palm or finger pad), and

aprosodia (analogue of aphasia affecting expression or comprehension of the emotional aspects of language, i.e. pitch, rhythm, intonation). Practically speaking, testing for these more esoteric deficits is not commonly part of the acute stroke evaluation, but may be helpful in confirming suspicion of non-dominant hemispheric ischemia.

★ **TIPS AND TRICKS**

Agnostic patients presents a unique challenge regarding consent for IV rt-PA as they may refute the need for treatment. One proposed method is to provide a "thought experiment." Ask the patient *hypothetically*, "If you were to have a devastating stroke, would you in that instance want to be treated knowing the risks and benefits of tPA as discussed?" An answer in the affirmative places the treating physician on more solid ethical ground in the acute setting [5].

Another cortical syndrome of clinical importance for bedside stroke diagnosis is visual field loss. Simplistically, the abrupt onset of homonymous hemianopsia is a posterior cerebral artery (PCA) or posterior MCA territory stroke until proven otherwise. Often, visual field cuts present as part of the collage of larger stroke syndromes, but may present in isolation with pure occipital lobe ischemia. Strokes affecting the optic radiations typically cause contralateral quandrantanopsias; temporal lobe ischemia involving the inferior optic radiations (i.e. Meyer's loop) typically affects the superior visual quadrant, as opposed to parietal lesions affecting the superior optic radiations and the inferior visual quadrant. Clinically, patients often do not recognize visual field loss unless confronted, but historical clues may include bumping into walls or merging into traffic. Rather than recognizing a lateralized deficit in both visual fields, patients more commonly complain of peripheral vision loss in the contalateral eye (easily teased out by confrontational testing at the bedside – see item 3 in the NIHSS). Treating patients with thrombolysis for isolated visual field loss is an individualized decision. While the NIHSS score indicates minor severity in these situations, a visual field deficit may nonetheless be severely disabling, particularly for patients who require good vision for employment or those that already have vision problems at baseline. As in all scenarios, an objective conversation with the stroke patient regarding risk and benefits of therapy will often guide one's hand.

> ★ TIPS AND TRICKS
>
> Lesions posterior to the optic chiasm (e.g. cerebral infarct) generate visual field defects that respect the vertical midline (i.e. hemianopsias), whereas those anterior the chiasm (e.g. branch retinal artery occlusion) respect the horizontal midline (i.e. altitudinal defect). Branch retinal artery occlusions may present as a *monocular* quadrantanopia.

Small vessel (lacunar) syndromes

Lacunar strokes include five classical syndromes, with some having multiple possible anatomic localizations (Table 1.3).

Table 1.3 The lacunar syndromes

Syndrome	Signs/symptoms	Localization	Vascular supply
Pure motor	Contralesional hemiparesis	Posterior limb of internal capsule, corona radiata or basis pontis	Lenticulostriate branches of the MCA or perforating arteries from the basilar artery
Pure sensory	Contralesional hemisensory loss	Ventroposterolateral nucleus of the thalamus	Lenticulostriate branches of the MCA or small thalamoperforators from the PCA
Sensorimotor	Contralesional weakness and numbness	Thalamus and adjacent posterior limb of internal capsule	Lenticulostriate branches from the MCA
Dysarthria–clumsy hand	Slurred speech and (typically fine motor) weakness of contralesional hand	Basis pontis, between rostral third and caudal two thirds	Perforating arteries from the basilar artery
Ataxia–hemiparesis	Contralesional (mild to moderate) hemiparesis and limb ataxia out of proportion to the degree of weakness	Posterior limb of internal capsule or basis pontis	Lenticulostriate branches of the MCA or perforating arteries from the basilar
Hemiballismus/hemichorea	Contralesional limb flailing or dyskinesias	Subthalamic nucleus	Perforating arteries from anterior choroidal (ICA), PCOM arteries

ICA, internal carotid artery; MCA, middle cerebral artery; PCA, posterior cerebral artery; PCOM, posterior communicating.

Table 1.4 The midbrain and medullary syndromes

Syndrome	Signs/symptoms	Localization	Vascular supply
Weber	Ipsilesional 3rd nerve palsy, contralesional hemiparesis (including the lower face)	Medial midbrain/ cerebral peduncle	Deep penetrating artery from PCA (see Table 1.1)
Benedikt	Ipsilesional 3rd nerve palsy, contralateral involuntary movements (intention tremor, hemichorea, or hemiathetosis)	Ventral midbrain involving red nucleus	Deep penetrating artery from PCA or paramedian penetrating branches of basilar artery
Nothnagel	Ipsilesional 3rd nerve palsy, contralesional dysmetria, and contralesional limb ataxia	Superior cerebellar peduncle	Deep penetrating artery from PCA
Wallenburg	Ipsilesional facial and contralesional body hypalgesia and thermoanesthesia, ipsilesional palatal weakness, dysphagia, dysarthria, nystagmus, vertigo, nausea/vomiting, ipsilesional Horner syndrome, skew deviation, singultus	Lateral medulla	PICA (should raise concern for disease in parent vertebral artery)
Dejerine	Ipsilesional tongue weakness and contralesional hemiparesis +/– contralesional loss of proprioception and vibratory sense	Medial medulla	Vertebral artery or anterior spinal artery

PCA, posterior cerebral artery; PICA, posterior inferior cerebellar artery.

- pure motor – contralateral hemiparesis; localizes to posterior limb of internal capsule, corona radiata, or basis pontis (ventral pons); secondary to occlusion of lenticulostriates branches of the MCA or perforating arteries from the basilar
- pure sensory – contralateral hemisensory deficit; localizes to ventroposterolateral nucleus of the thalamus secondary to lenticulostriates or small thalamoperforators from the PCA
- sensorimotor – contralateral paresis and numbness; localizes to thalamus and adjacent posterior limb of internal capsule (thalamocapsular)
- dysarthria – clumsy hand – slurred speech and weakness of contralateral hand usually most evident when writing or performing other fine motor tasks (may also include supranuclear facial weakness, tongue deviation, and dysphagia), localizes to basis pontis between upper third and lower two-thirds
- ataxic hemiparesis – contralateral mild to moderate hemiparesis and limb ataxia out of proportion to the degree of weakness, usually affecting the leg more than the arm, localizes to posterior limb of internal capsule or basis pontis

- there is a rare sixth lacunar syndrome presenting with contralateral hemichorea or hemiballismus from a small infarct in the basal ganglia or subthalamic nucleus.

✋ CAUTION

Lacunar strokes typically present with fluctuating symptoms in the acute period. The so-called "capsular warning syndrome" often presents with oscillating sensorimotor deficits over a 24 to 48-hour period representing a small lenticulostriate perforator artery in the process of occlusion. In too many cases, tPA treatment is withheld due to "rapidly improving symptoms" in the hyperacute period only to find the patient with a dense hemiparesis the following morning secondary to completed small vessel stroke.

Brainstem syndromes

There are several vertebrobasilar brainstem syndromes that should be recognizable in the acute stroke setting. These are often caused by occlusion of a small brainstem-penetrating artery stemming from a larger parent vessel, and can therefore be related to either large artery atherosclerosis or small vessel occlusive disease. Less commonly, a micro-embolus may find its way into one of these perfora-tors, but this is difficult to distinguish without a source of embolus. Named midbrain and medullary syndromes are described in Table 1.4.

Pontine syndromes (see Table 1.1 – basilar territory stroke) are often caused by occlusion of deep or circumferential pontine penetrating branch arteries in the presence of a patent basilar artery. A hallmark of deep pontine infarcts is an abnormality of horizontal gaze and dysarthria. A chief complaint is horizontal diplopia, and presenting signs may include ipsilateral lateral gaze palsy from involve-ment of the abucens nucleus (CN VI) or as an inter-nuclear ophthalmoplegia (INO) from injury to the medial longitudinal fasciculus that yokes conjugate horizontal gaze – although the latter is consistently seen in paramedian midbrain syndromes as well. Due to proximity of the abducens nucleus to CN VII, these patients may also have a peripheral pattern of facial weakness involving upper and lower facial muscles ipsilateral to the infarct. Involvement of more ventral portions of the pons (i.e. corticospinal and corticopontocerebellar tracts) causes contra-lateral hemiparesis or ataxia.

> ★ TIPS AND TRICKS
>
> If a patient presents with neck pain and/or Horner's syndrome, particularly in young adults, consider cervical artery dissection. Vertebral artery dissection often presents with ipsilesional lateral medullary syndrome and/or cerebellar stroke due to posterior inferior cerebellar artery (PICA) territory infarction. Distal carotid artery dissection may cause lower cranial nerve palsies, but this is a false localizer for brainstem stroke.

> ☝ CAUTION
>
> Be vigilant of the "locked-in" patient; that is a patient who may appear *comatose* but yet has voluntary blinking or vertical eye movements allowing bedside communication. Locked-in

syndrome is caused by bilateral ventral pontine injury with preserved rostral brainstem function including spared level of consciousness from an intact reticular activating system and vertical gaze centers in the midbrain. Similar to top of the basilar syndrome mentioned above, recognizing a devastating pattern of brainstem dysfunction in the acute stroke setting requires immediate evaluation of the basilar artery for possible reperfusion therapy.

Stroke versus TIA?

Transient ischemic attacks (TIA) occur in approxi-mately 15% of patients before an eventual stroke, with the highest risk in the first days to weeks fol-lowing an event [6,7]. While TIAs do not always come to medical attention, their presentation in the acute stroke setting ostensibly complicates the treatment decision in patients who may be exhibit-ing some improvement. The majority of TIAs resolve in less than 60 minutes whereas the majority of true strokes reach peak deficit in the same time frame. A 2009 scientific statement from the American Heart Association/American Stroke Association discour-ages the use of traditional time-based definitions of TIA in favor of a *tissue-based* definition (i.e. the presence or absence of lesions on diffusion-weighted MR imaging) [8]. The fact that 30–50% of TIAs will result in diffusion-weighted abnormalities on brain MRI emphasizes the importance of making a *clinical* diagnosis in the acute setting. The diag-nosis of a TIA requires absolute resolution of symp-toms, whereas a persistent deficit should continue to raise concern for a treatable stroke. If a patient returns completely to their neurological baseline (100%), then the clock starts over and any recurrent deficits may be considered a new event (i.e. *reopen-ing* the treatment window). Evaluation of TIA in the acute stroke setting also requires some assessment of risk. A common practice at US stroke centers is to admit patients following TIA in order to expedite the urgent workup of causative mechanisms, including noninvasive vascular imaging and cardiac evaluation. The ABCD2 score has been established as a validated clinical tool to aid in risk assessment and management decisions [9] (Table 1.5). The AHA/ASA statement referenced above provides the

Table 1.5 The ABCD2 score

Age	>60 years	1 point
Blood pressure	≥140/90 mmHg	1 point
Clinical features	Other than below	0 points
	Speech disturbance without weakness	1 point
	Unilateral weakness	2 points
Duration	<10 minutes	0 points
	10–59 minutes	1 point
	≥60 minutes	2 points
Diabetes	Present	1 point

following recommendation as a possible algorithm in the acute setting:

"It is reasonable to hospitalize patients with TIA if they present within 72 hours of the event and any of the following criteria are present":

a. ABCD2 score of ≥3
b. ABCD2 score of 0 to 2 and uncertainty that diagnostic workup can be completed within 2 days as an outpatient
c. ABCD2 score of 0 to 2 and other evidence that indicates the patient's event was caused by focal ischemia.

Stroke mimics

Of the many judgments required of the stroke physician at the bedside during an emergency, perhaps the most difficult is consideration of the stroke mimic. As treatment with rt-PA clearly is not without risk it is important that the physician be able to rapidly differentiate a stroke mimic from symptoms due to retinal, hemispheric, or brainstem ischemia. The following paragraphs highlight frequently encountered stroke mimics and how to more reliably differentiate them from ischemic stroke in the bedside evaluation.

Following a seizure, postictal focal neurological deficit can appear identical to any cortical stroke syndrome, and without a reliable history or eyewitness can be nearly impossible to diagnose prospectively. One would hope that the seizure patient would be able to provide a telling history but this often is not the case, particularly in encephalopathic or aphasic patients when the ictal event is unwitnessed. The most commonly encountered

postictal phenomenon is Todd's paralysis (postictal hemiparesis), but the bedside physician should be aware that almost any focal cortical neurological deficit can be witnessed following a seizure depending on the anatomic location of the seizure focus. Examples include postictal aphasia, sensory disturbance, and neglect. While seizure at the outset of symptoms is a *relative* contraindication to rt-PA, it should be noted that focal seizures can often herald ischemic stroke onset, particularly of cardioembolic origin. In cases of high suspicion for stroke, attention should be made to the bedside exam and head CT for diagnostic confirmation before ruling out treatment options.

★ TIPS AND TRICKS

Gaze preference may help differentiate seizure versus stroke – in a large MCA stroke, eyes will deviate towards the lesion, i.e. away from the side of paralysis. In an ongoing seizure, eyes will deviate away from the ictus, i.e. towards the side of focal motor tonic–clonic activity. Gaze may reverse preference in the postictal state, looking away from Todd's paralysis.

Another common mimic that can be difficult to diagnose is migraine with aura. The migraine patient, of course, typically will have an associated headache most often following the onset of focal neurological symptoms. However, this is not always the case. Older individuals, in particular, are prone to migraine equivalents without head pain, making the diagnosis even more difficult as this population is typically also at a higher risk for stroke. Like seizures, migraine equivalents can mimic almost any focal cortical neurological deficit due to the spreading cortical depression that is characteristic of migraine pathology. A history of migraine, as well as the presence of commonly associated symptoms of nausea, anorexia, photophobia, phonophobia, and positive visual phenomenon, can be helpful. Other clues include a temporal "marching" quality of symptoms (i.e. from face to arm to leg) and positive symptoms such as parasthesias. However, it should be emphasized that the diagnosis of migraine in the acute stroke patient, particularly in persons with legitimate vascular risk factors, remains a diagnosis of exclusion. Hemorrhagic strokes and some less common causes of ischemic stroke, such as reversible cerebral vasoconstriction syndrome and carotid dissection, may be associated with acute headache at the time of the event.

Metabolic derangements that may mimic stroke include hyper- or hypoglycemia, electrolyte disturbances, or infection. It is widely held that any metabolic stress on the body can cause "stroke reactivation" or "anamnestic syndrome." In this case, symptoms of a prior stroke from which a patient has recovered can re-emerge as the metabolic stress on the brain increases. A history of identical symptoms during a prior ischemic event or evidence of chronic infarction in a relevant vascular territory on noncontrast head CT can help make this diagnosis. Generally, neurological symptoms improve in parallel with correction of infectious/ metabolic derangement.

Multiple sclerosis (MS) may mimic almost any other neurological disorder, including stroke. MS tends to present in middle-aged women, sometimes with history of other autoimmune disease. MS flares tend to have a "crescendo–decrescendo" character and if a careful history is taken, symptoms rarely are at their most severe at onset, as is the case in stroke. Isolated acute demyelinating lesions may also show restricted diffusion on brain MRI, often difficult to distinguish from acute infarct without corroborating history and exam.

A mass lesion may mimic stroke but generally will present with headache, which is classically positional (worse with lying down or with Valsalva maneuvers), and nausea/vomiting. Symptoms in this case are likely to be gradual in onset; however, hemorrhagic metastases can produce acute neurological changes and seizure as well.

Peripheral vertigo may be very difficult to distinguish from ischemia in the posterior circulation. Helpful characteristics in identifying central vertigo are vertical nystagmus, nystagmus that changes direction with change in gaze, and neighborhood brainstem signs and symptoms (e.g. diplopia, dysphagia, dysarthria). A positive Dix–Hallpike test or head thrust maneuver may suggest a peripheral etiology, though, ultimately, a patient with a high-risk vascular profile and acute vertigo must immediately raise the clinician's concern for stroke. Notably, medial branch PICA territory infarctions in midline cerebellar structures often present with isolated acute vestibular syndrome.

Occasionally, isolated limb weakness or numbness is caused by a peripheral lesion (e.g. foot drop from peroneal compression, arm weakness from cervical disc disease) and will mimic stroke. Peripheral causes of weakness or sensory disturbance are usually excluded by a careful examination. A practical example includes the "Saturday night" radial nerve palsy causing wrist drop that may mimic cortical hand syndrome from a stroke in the lateral precentral gyrus or "hand knob." In peripheral wrist drop, supporting the wrist will reveal intact strength of intrinsic hand muscles as opposed to a cortical hand syndrome.

Probably the most common stroke mimics reflect somatization or conversion disorder. These patients are especially difficult to diagnose, commonly presenting with hemiparesis/hemiplegia, unilateral sensory disturbance, or speech arrest. Functional aphasia is generally relatively easy to detect by an experienced examiner, as these patients can present with stuttering speech rather than lack of fluency, or will be slow to respond to questions without having any legitimate word-finding difficulty or comprehensive errors.

★ TIPS AND TRICKS

True expressive aphasia should also involve agraphia; the inability to speak with preserved ability to communicate through writing is characteristically not consistent with physiological aphasia.

Functional hemiparesis may be challenging to distinguish, but there are some relatively straightforward bedside maneuvers that can aid in the diagnosis. Examples include the Hoover sign, observation of upper extremity drift without pronation, and effort-dependent and break-away weakness. Subjective numbness in a nonanatomic pattern is another clue. For example, inability to detect vibration over the left side of the frontal bone while vibratory sense remains intact over the right is not a physiological deficit. The subjectivity of sensory symptoms makes some vascular neurologists hesitant to offer treatment in these cases, though it should be pointed out that thalamic stroke can present with a true hemisensory deficit.

🔬 SCIENCE REVISITED

In a review of 512 consecutive cases treated with IV rt-PA within 3 hours of symptom onset, 21% were found not to have an infarct on follow-up imaging. The most common stroke mimics encountered included seizure, complicated migraine, and somatization. More importantly, there were no instances of symptomatic intracerebral hemorrhage, emphasizing the minimal risk of treatment in this group [10]. If suspicion for ischemic stroke exists, one should not withhold treatment simply for fear of a mimic.

The history – guessing the age of a stroke and more

Once the neurologist suspects that an acute stroke *is* the cause of the patient's symptoms, the next immediate question to be answered is whether that patient is appropriate for treatment. The critical factor in this determination is frequently the most difficult – the exact time when the patient was *last known well*. This seems fairly straightforward, but in practice it can be challenging. The physician is often very clearly told when the patient was *first known unwell* but this point is somewhat irrelevant. For consideration of treatment within recommended time windows, the clock starts when the patient was last known to be symptom free. A substantial proportion of patients are alone when their stroke symptoms begin, and if they are unable to provide a clear, cogent history the physician must obtain that detail of the history from whomever saw them last. This is important particularly in patients who awaken with their symptoms.

🔬 SCIENCE REVISITED

A number of published stroke registries in the 1970s–1980s found an early to midmorning predominance in onset of ischemic stroke, potentially coinciding with diurnal peaks in blood pressure and cortisol. Unfortunately, many stroke patients wake up with their symptoms, making any determination of a time of onset difficult [11]. Research is underway to determine the safety and efficacy of treating wakeup stroke with thrombolysis.

Unless the patient awoke at some point during the night and was clearly asymptomatic (e.g. able to ambulate to the bathroom or speak to their spouse, but now aphasic and hemiparetic), the window for treatment, by definition, would begin when they were last known well – in this case, the evening before, prior to going asleep.

★ TIPS AND TRICKS

Witnesses do not often volunteer this information, so it is important to investigate such things as nighttime awakenings, possible phone conversations (check their mobile phone for recent calls), evidence of normal activity such as shopping receipts, or potential witnesses who regularly interact with a patient found down. Searching a purse or wallet from Jane or John Doe stroke patients may provide crucial clues or contact information that could lead to treatment.

Once the time the patient was last known well is firmly established, there are several other key pieces of basic medical information that should be attained on arrival for evaluation of the acute stroke patient. The patient's blood pressure and blood sugar are important, as are the ranges of each that are considered appropriate for treatment with IV rt-PA. A blood pressure of more than 185/110 mmHg that is not correctable is considered an absolute contraindication to treatment; considering this early in the acute evaluation will save time when the rt-PA is ready. Serum glucose of less than 50 mg/dL or greater than 400 mg/dL is also a contraindication, as this may suggest the presence of a mimic. If possible to attain, a brief past medical history is essential. Particularly important is the consideration of a potential stroke patient's vascular risk profile: history of hypertension, diabetes, hyperlipidemia, smoking, atrial fibrillation, and of course, prior stroke or TIA. While clearly none of the above is required to diagnose stroke and the absence of risk factors should not preclude treatment if suspicion for stroke is high, weighing a patient's risk can help tip the scales when making a swift judgment about whether or not to administer rt-PA in an unclear case. A quick review of a patient's medication list is helpful. Not only can a medication list give clues as to prior medical history, but also the presence of warfarin or other anticoagulation adds a significant factor to be weighed in the ultimate decision to treat (more below in the laboratory section).

Rapid examination of the acute stroke patient

After obtaining a clear understanding of the initial presentation with particular attention to when the patient was last known well, a focused medical history, and a brief review of medications, the physician should move to the focused physical examination. In the rapid evaluation of acute stroke, this exam is essentially the NIH stroke scale (see Chapter 9 Appendix). This 11-item examination was designed as a research tool to quickly and consistently measure stroke severity; however, since the report of the NINDS tPA study, it has become mainstream clinical practice in the acute stroke setting. The NIHSS contains selected elements commonly affected in acute stroke syndromes including evaluation of mental status, cranial nerves, visuospatial, motor, sensory, and cerebellar function and can be performed by the experienced examiner in roughly 5 to 10 minutes. By the completion of the NIHSS, the physician should have a reasonable idea of whether the patient is having a stroke, the severity of the deficit, and the localization of the lesion in the nervous system. The scale is designed such that the higher the score, the more severe the neurological impairment, with scores ranging from 0 to 42. Minor strokes, such as those caused by small emboli, are generally considered in the range of 0–4 points, with large artery strokes caused by proximal vascular occlusions producing symptoms commonly exceeding 10 points.

While the NIHSS is a rapid and fairly consistent screening tool, one should be aware of its limitations. For example, the scale will differentially rate ischemic lesions of identical volume depending on the hemispheric location. A complete, proximal left middle cerebral artery occlusion will generate an NIHSS score in the 22–25 range, whereas the same proximal occlusion in the right MCA territory will give a score closer to 15. This is due to the fact that aphasia is given more weight than neglect in the scoring paradigm. If the physician is concerned about a lesion in the nondominant parietal lobe, an insult that is commonly unrecognized as a stroke, evaluating the patient for agraphesthesia and stereoagnosia is not only appropriate but may well be more helpful than any part of the NIHSS. There are some strokes that do not register any points on the scale. Examples are the embolic stroke affecting the portion of the motor strip that controls hand or finger movements, or the midline cerebellar stroke affecting gait but not limb ataxia. Small lacunar strokes in the posterior fossa can cause isolated vertigo that can be extremely disabling but could still register no score on the NIHSS. A low score (even 0) on the NIHSS should not, by default, defer the physician from considering treatment. While the NIHSS is a validated, rapid way to evaluate the function of the nervous system, it originated as a measure of stroke severity for clinical trials and is not meant to be a substitute for a thorough neurological exam.

Beyond the NIHSS and other focused neurological examination, there are a number of general physical findings that are useful in evaluation of the acute stroke patient. Vital signs, especially blood pressure, are of particular interest. Not only does hypertension at presentation convey an increased risk of stroke but, as was previously mentioned, the administration of rt-PA requires blood pressure of less than 185/110 mmHg. Complicating matters further is that rapid lowering of blood pressure in the acute stroke patient can actually be detrimental due to its deleterious effects on cerebral perfusion.

Auscultation of cardiac and carotid sounds can be beneficial in some cases, as can palpation of peripheral pulses. An irregularly irregular cardiac rhythm, for example, may indicate atrial fibrillation, which may provide a substrate for cardioembolism. A patient with stroke symptoms, chest pain, and asymmetric radial pulses may have a thoracic aortic dissection or aneurysm, which is a vascular surgical emergency and should prompt additional vascular imaging of the chest and neck in addition to head CT. Pupillary asymmetry can be another helpful observation, though not a formal part of the NIHSS. In a young patient presenting with neck pain and stroke symptoms, miosis and partial ptosis are signs of Horner's syndrome, often associated with carotid dissection due to disruption of the ascending cervical sympathetic chain. Lastly, while also not a part of the NIHSS, eliciting muscle stretch reflexes for upper motor signs (i.e. hyperreflexia, clonus, Babinski sign) may be useful in distinguishing central from peripheral causes of weakness (keeping in mind that in the acute setting, the stroke patient may well present with normoactive reflexes).

Diagnostic data

The all important head CT

After collection of a brief history and execution of a focused, screening neurological examination, the physician should have an idea regarding the likelihood that the patient is to be offered emergent treatment for his/her symptoms. The next step is to obtain a stat noncontrast CT of the head. It is obligate that this study be obtained prior to the delivery of any treatment for acute stroke in order to rule out intracerebral hemorrhage (ICH).

> ☆ **TIPS AND TRICKS**
>
> Acute hemorrhage is hyperdense on head CT; other hyperdense findings on CT include calcification (choroid plexus, pineal gland, basal ganglia), intravenous contrast, bone, and metallic materials such as endovascular aneurysm coils or shrapnel. Hyperdensity can be measured in Hounsfield units and can be used by the experienced neuroradiologist to differentiate acute hemorrhage from calcifications.

While acute ischemic stroke and ICH may have virtually the same clinical presentation, some historical features can be a clue to the latter such as more prominent headache, uncontrolled hypertension, more abrupt signs of increased intracranial pressure, or a known coagulopathy. Nevertheless, these entities are clinically similar enough to warrant CT imaging in all cases where diagnostic differentiation is necessary. Current AHA/ASA and JCAHO guidelines recommend an interval of no more than 20 minutes between patient arrival and initiation of head CT. While it is not required that all physicians treating acute stroke be neuroradiological experts, it is beneficial to appreciate certain corroborative signs of ischemic stroke on the noncontrast head CT. The most commonly observed radiological signature of large vessel occlusions is the hyperdense artery sign. For MCA occlusions, this will appear as a dense proximal M1 segment at the base of the brain ipsilateral to a clinical hemispheric syndrome.

> ☆ **TIPS AND TRICKS**
>
> Dehydration or calcific atherosclerosis may cause arteries to look hyperdense on CT; the key is to compare the dense artery with the contralateral side. If both sides are "dense," consider one of the above radiological mimics and whether the imaging fits with the clinical presentation.

While the dense artery sign is most often observed when there is acute thrombus in the proximal MCA, it is also a diagnostic sign of basilar artery occlusion. The latter, while easily recognized by the trained radiological eye, is frequently missed by the bedside examiner due to the often less-clear picture of brainstem ischemia.

> ☝ **CAUTION**
>
> In the comatose patient being evaluated for acute stroke, pay close attention for the dense basilar artery sign indicating "top of the basilar" or "locked-in" syndrome. These are devastating ischemic events necessitating immediate reperfusion efforts.

Another early ischemic change appreciated on head CT is the loss of the "insular ribbon," or the loss of gray–white differentiation in the cortex secondary to ischemia from MCA occlusion. This is best appreciated in contrast to the opposite hemisphere with normal perfusion. This is particularly important when trying to appreciate the size or age of an infarct. When the time of stroke onset is unclear, a marked hypodensity may indicate an infarct is older than a few hours. Early ischemic changes encompassing greater than one-third the MCA territory likely represents sizable infarct of great severity, and may be a poor prognostic factor for late attempts at reperfusion.

> ☆ **TIPS AND TRICKS**
>
> Head positioning within the CT scanner should be accounted for; a head positioned askew in the CT gantry can result in the false appearance of cortical asymmetries.

Though all of these signs can be seen in the acute stroke evaluation, the absence of clear evidence of stroke on the CT scan should not discourage treatment – in fact, except in those cases mentioned above, the head CT in the acute stroke setting may well be entirely unremarkable.

Laboratory and ancillary studies

While the physician is obtaining a history, performing a neurological examination, and reviewing the head CT, blood should have been obtained from the patient and been delivered to the laboratory with results pending. As emphasis, it is of vital importance that blood be collected and sent to the lab shortly after the patient arrives to the emergency department and certainly before travel to the imaging suite. This is important because of the potential need to review laboratory results prior to administration of thrombolytic. Blood glucose must be obtained prior to treating with IV tPA. Many patients can be treated prior to final lab results if there is no clinical reason to anticipate an abnormality. During the typical stroke alert, complete blood count, basic metabolic panel, and coagulation profile should be sent at a minimum. If a patient reports warfarin as a home medication, the physician *must* know the INR prior to initiating treatment with rt-PA. In the NINDS tPA trial, any patient was excluded for rt-PA if warfarin had been taken in the previous 24 hours. However, the FDA stipulated excluding treatment only for an INR >1.7. This criterion varies across centers and ultimately it falls on the physician to make a best judgment of risk over benefit, and hence the reason a quick but thorough review of past medical history and the patient's home medications is crucial in the early stages of evaluation. The most likely reason a patient with atrial fibrillation on warfarin presents with acute stroke is secondary to a subtherapeutic INR. Other important data to review before treatment with IV rt-PA are PTT (in cases where heparin has been used in the last 24 hours) and a platelet count >100,000/μL.

Additionally, the recent approval and growing usage of nonwarfarin anticoagulants for stroke prevention in atrial fibrillation – including the direct thrombin inhibitor, dabigatran, and factor Xa inhibitor, rivaroxaban – may not reveal an abnormal coagulation profile in all cases. Therefore, it is vital to know the current medications for stroke patients with atrial fibrillation being considered for tPA, independent of laboratory data.

★ TIPS AND TRICKS

For patients with severe symptoms who are outside the window of treatment for IV rt-PA and being considered for interventional therapy, the glomerular filtration rate (GFR) indicates risk of renal complications with IV contrast. However, most centers consider acute stroke a sufficient emergency as to allow the administration of IV contrast without explicit knowledge of the GFR. Despite regular use of angiographic imaging, contrast nephropathy is surprisingly uncommon in the acute stroke setting.

Along with phlebotomy, establishing intravenous access immediately upon patient arrival and prior to travel to CT is also crucial, both so that the rt-PA bolus may be administered immediately upon determination of its indication and in order to deliver intravenous contrast in the event that angiographic imaging is required. This is not only of clinical import, but also may be an obstacle to recommended door-to-CT time, particularly in older patients with difficult venous access.

The final piece of data that should not be forgotten during the acute stroke evaluation is the electrocardiogram (ECG). Acute stroke and myocardial infarction often coincide and the latter should not be overlooked when focused on the management of the former. Acute coronary syndrome can also cause acute neurological deficits, generally as a result of cerebral hypoperfusion that is unmasked during an episode of relative hypotension. Many stroke centers include serum troponin among the laboratory studies that are routinely sent during the initial evaluation. In the case of acute myocardial infarction presenting with neurological deficit, rapid support of the cardiovascular system is vital. In the unstable patient, addressing cardiorespiratory status is the foremost priority regardless of the neurological condition.

Biomarkers in acute stroke diagnosis?

In addition to advances in neuroimaging, avid research is underway to establish a serum biomarker for acute stroke diagnosis, the so-called "stroke troponin." Numerous individual proteins and protein panels have been studied, including such markers as N-methyl D-aspartate (NMDA) receptor antibodies, metalloproteinases, and von Willibrand's factor, but lack appropriate specificity to distinguish ischemic stroke from other brain injury or vascular disease [12]. Gene expression profiles offer the promise of greater specificity. In 2006, Tang and colleagues demonstrated that RNA transcribed by serum leukocytes could derive a gene expression profile distinguishing patients with acute ischemic stroke from normal controls with sensitivity 89% and specificity 100%, and later validated this 18-gene panel in a larger cohort achieving sensitivity/specificity of 93/95%. A separate analysis by Barr et al., using a different microarray chip, reported similar results with a nine-gene panel deriving five of the same genes [12]. The promise of RNA expression analysis has been further demonstrated in distinguishing ischemic stroke subtypes in the acute setting, which might help tailor diagnostic and treatment pathways. While this area of research is exciting, external validation in larger cohorts is required before translation to clinical care can be reached. Beyond serving as a tool in ischemic stroke diagnosis, other potential applications of serum biomarkers in the acute stroke setting include prediction of ischemic penumbra, estimation of infarct volume, and correlation to eventual outcome.

The decision to treat

After diagnosis of acute stroke, appraisal of radiographic and laboratory data, and careful review of exclusion criteria for rt-PA, the physician should be prepared to offer treatment. In general, IV rt-PA is considered an emergent therapy and patient consent is not mandatorily required although individual hospitals may apply this exception to the requirement for informed consent differently. Use of presumed consent in emergency situations is particularly relevant for aphasic or encephalopathic stroke patients where communication is challenging and the need for treatment is imminent. However, in most situations a discussion with the patient or their family prior to treatment is prudent and requires the physician be knowledgeable of the risks and benefits of therapy – discussed in detail in the chapter on stroke therapeutics. The points to be covered are relatively straightforward, but time is a major concern so balance in addressing the important details without dwelling on minutiae is important. By this point, the physician should already have ordered IV rt-PA from the pharmacy and be ready to retrieve it once the decision to treat

is made. Additionally, communication with the nursing staff during this time is essential for rapid administration of treatment: IV access should be ensured, an infusion pump should be at the bedside, and close BP monitoring should meet parameters less than 185/110 mmHg (i.e. treat with IV labetalol pushes, nicardipine drip as needed).

The last thing that should be done prior to pushing the IV rt-PA bolus is a final pretreatment assessment of the NIHSS. This can be brief and focused, but the examiner needs to ensure the persistence and consistency of the deficit. While rapidly improving or minor symptoms are a relative contraindication to treatment in the listed exclusion criteria, this should be considered in the context of each given case. As aforementioned, the physician and patient can consider the perceived disability if the deficits prior to treatment were to persist with no further improvement. Stroke symptoms (particularly in small vessel occlusions) can often fluctuate, so the bedside exam most proximate to the moment of treatment is ultimately the most reliable. Again, one should not withhold treatment for minor improvements in the neurological exam, particularly when the patient is not returning to baseline.

⚙ SCIENCE REVISITED

Treatment of acute ischemic stroke is time-dependent, and receiving IV tPA is the most important factor associated with favorable outcomes other than the severity of the stroke itself. Pooled analysis from the NINDS rt-PA, ECASS, and ATLANTIS clinical stroke trials reveal the odds of a favorable outcome decrease with every extended minute from onset to treatment with tPA [13]. These minutes of delay equate to worse outcomes in stroke manifesting as increased long-term disability and death. The AHA/ASA's GWTG program recommends door-to-needle (i.e. IV tPA) time of ≤60 minutes, a goal achieved in less than one-third of all ischemic stroke patients treated in the US [3]. Yet, the concept of "ultraearly" stroke treatment has been realized by a group from the Helsinki University Central Hospital who published a simple protocol in 2012 achieving median door-to-needle times of *20 minutes* [14].

Conclusion

Clearly, this chapter cannot fully encompass the spectrum of ideas, opinions, and evidence that guide the evaluation of the acute stroke patient, nor does it highlight the entirety of hard work and ongoing research dedicated to improving the current provision of acute stroke care. Nevertheless, the principles are universal: acute brain ischemia is the downstream result of often-chronic disease where physicians and provider teams have the ability to most immediately impact a stroke patient's life and future abilities. The ultimate goal of any acute stroke protocol in the current age is to rapidly establish the time of symptom onset, make an accurate bedside diagnosis, and administer reperfusion therapy to eligible patients; yet it is the providers and patients themselves that enable the achievement of quality and effective care and all together should continue to herald the charge, "time is brain."

Selected bibliography

1. The National Institute of Neurological Disorders and Stroke rt-PA Stroke Study Group. Tissue plasminogen activator for acute ischemic stroke. *N Engl J Med* 1995; **333**: 1581–7.
2. Agency for Healthcare Research and Quality, USDoHaHS. *National Guideline Clearinghouse.* Available at: http://www.guideline.gov/ (accessed August 2012).
3. Fonarow GC, Smith EE, Saver JL, et al. Timeliness of tissue-type plasminogen activator therapy in acute ischemic stroke: patient characteristics, hospital factors, and outcomes associated with door-to-needle times within 60 minutes. *Circulation* 2011; **123**: 750–8.
4. Brazis PW, Masdeu JC, Biller B. *Localization in Clinical Neurology*, 5th edition. Philadelphia, PA: Lippincott, Williams, & Wilkins–Wolters Kluwer, 2007.
5. Worrall BB, Chen DT, Dimberg EL. Correspondence: Should thrombolysis be given to a stroke patient refusing therapy due to profound anosagnosia? *Neurology* 2005; **65**: 500.
6. Roger VL, Go AS, Lloyd-Jones DM, et al. Heart disease and stroke statistics – 2012 update: a report from the American Heart Association. *Circulation* 2012; **125**: e2–e220.
7. Johnston SC, Gress DR, Browner WS, Sidney S. Short-term prognosis after emergency department diagnosis of TIA. *JAMA* 2000; **284**: 2901–6.
8. Easton JD, Saver JL, Albers GW, et al. Definition and evaluation of transient ischemic attack: a scientific statement for healthcare professionals from the American Heart Association/American Stroke Association Stroke Council; Council on Cardiovascular Surgery and Anesthesia; Council on Cardiovascular Radiology and Intervention; Council on Cardiovascular Nursing; and the Interdisciplinary Council on Peripheral Vascular Disease. The American Academy of Neurology affirms the value of this statement as an educational tool for neurologists. *Stroke* 2009; **40**: 2276–93.
9. Johnston SC, Rothwell PM, Nguyen-Huynh MN, et al. Validation and refinement of scores to predict very early stroke risk after transient ischaemic attack. *Lancet* 2007; **369**: 283–92.
10. Chernyshev OY, Martin-Schild S, Albright KC, et al. Safety of tPA in stroke mimics and neuroimaging-negative cerebral ischemia. *Neurology* 2010; **74**: 1340–5.
11. Marler JR, Price TR, Clark GL, et al. Morning increase in onset of ischemic stroke. *Stroke* 1989; **20**: 473–6.
12. Jickling GC, Sharp FR. Blood biomarkers of ischemic stroke. *Neurotherapeutics* 2011; **8**: 349–60.
13. Hacke W, Donnan G, Fieschi C, et al. Association of outcome with early stroke treatment: pooled analysis of ATLANTIS, ECASS, and NINDS rt-PA stroke trials. *Lancet* 2004; **363**: 768–74.
14. Meretoja A, Strbian D, Mustanoja S, et al. Reducing in-hospital delay to 20 minutes in stroke thrombolysis. *Neurology* 2012; **79**: 306–13.

Neurovascular Imaging of the Acute Stroke Patient

Karthik Arcot, MD,[1] Jason M. Johnson, MD,[2] Michael H. Lev, MD,[2] and Albert J. Yoo, MD[2]

[1] Lutheran Medical Center, Brooklyn, NY
[2] Massachusetts General Hospital and Harvard Medical School, Boston, MA

Introduction

Neurology is undergoing a revolution in terms of understanding disease mechanisms and therapeutics, fueled in large part by the rapid advances in neuroimaging. Nowhere is this more true than in the field of stroke. While prevention remains the best intervention, the stroke burden related to the growing elderly population necessitates accurate diagnosis and triage to effective treatments for patients presenting with acute symptoms. This process is critically dependent on neuroimaging [1].

Advanced imaging techniques improve the delivery of emergency stroke care. Current acute treatments for stroke are predicated on time. Many acute ischemic stroke patients do not arrive in the narrow time window during which intravenous (IV) tissue plasminogen activator (tPA) can be safely administered. By depicting an individual patient's cerebrovascular physiology, neuroimaging may allow a more rational delivery of stroke therapies to patients who may benefit but are outside of current time windows. It can also identify patients who will benefit from catheter-based therapies. This is an active area of clinical research.

For these reasons, physicians who treat stroke patients must be familiar with the most common neuroimaging techniques. To this end, this chapter will provide a clinically relevant framework for neurovascular imaging of the acute stroke patient.

Technical considerations

Noncontrast computed tomography (NCCT) scan

CT scanning is based on the principle that tissues of varying densities attenuate X-rays to different degrees. This differential attenuation is converted to a gray-scale image of the body part being scanned. An arbitrary number, known as the CT Hounsfield unit (HU), is used to quantify these differences in tissue density with distilled water defined at zero HU. Using this system, air has a CT number of minus (−) 1000 HU and dense bone has a CT number of approximately plus (+) 1000 HU (Figure 2.1a).

Given its widespread availability, head NCCT is the predominant method for acute stroke imaging in the vast majority of medical centers. The major advantage is rapid and accurate diagnosis of intracranial hemorrhage, which appears hyperdense (i.e. brighter) relative to brain parenchyma (Figure 2.1a). Current guidelines recommend head NCCT as the only form of neuroimaging necessary to determine eligibility for IV tPA. The scan time is on the order of seconds (approximately 10–15 seconds per scan), and the images are instantly available for review at the scanner console.

The relative disadvantage of NCCT is its limited sensitivity (20–75%) and poor interobserver reliability for detecting acute ischemic changes in the hyperacute treatment window (e.g. within 3 to 6 hours of onset). Early ischemic changes include

Stroke, First Edition. Edited by Kevin M. Barrett and James F. Meschia.
© 2013 John Wiley & Sons, Ltd. Published 2013 by John Wiley & Sons, Ltd.

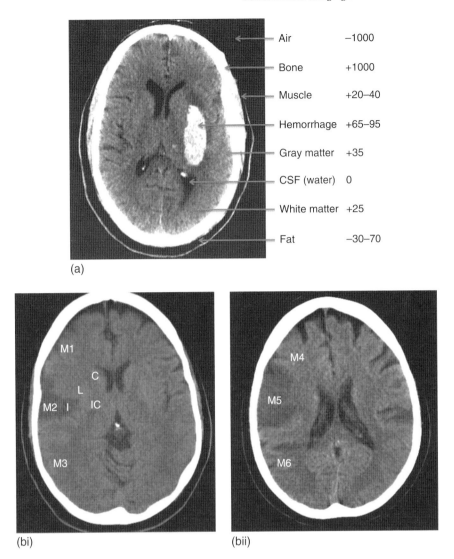

(a)

(bi)   (bii)

Figure 2.1 (a) Approximate average CT numbers (in Hounsfield Units, HU) of tissues routinely visualized on head CT scans (all typically ±5–10 HU). (bi) Sample Alberta Stroke Program Early CT Score (ASPECTS) grading system for ischemic hypodensity on unenhanced head CT, at the level of the basal ganglia. C, caudate head; IC, internal capsule; L, lenticular nuclei; I, insular cortex; M1, inferior frontal territory; M2, anterior temporal territory; M3, posterior temporal territory. An ischemic hypodensity is seen in the right M2 and I regions. (bii) Sample ASPECTS grading system for ischemic hypodensity on unenhanced head CT, at the level of the superior lateral ventricles (approximately 2 cm above basal ganglia level). M4, anterior superior frontal territory; M5, posterior superior frontal territory; M6, parietal territory. An ischemic hypodensity is seen in the right M5 region.

parenchymal hypoattenuation and focal cortical swelling (Figure 2.2a). In more well-established strokes, vasogenic edema may produce effacement of the CSF spaces, including the sulci, cisterns, and ventricles. Parenchymal hypoattenuation is related to increased water content from vasogenic edema and appears to be a sign of irreversible tissue injury, while recent studies suggest that focal swelling alone may be reversible. A 1% increase in tissue water corresponds to a 2–3 HU decrease in tissue density. In order to detect these subtle changes, use of narrow window width settings is recommended

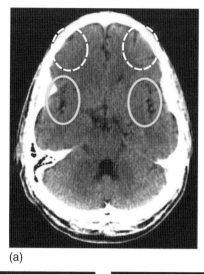

(a)

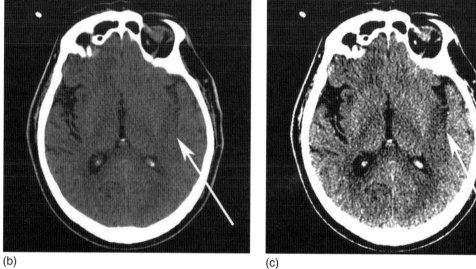

(b)   (c)

Figure 2.2 (a) Unenhanced CT signs of early stroke – the "insular ribbon" sign and "sulcal effacement."
The solid ellipses show portions of the insular cortices with subtle right (versus left) sided low attenuation
and loss of gray–white differentiation, secondary to early cytotoxic/vasogenic edema. The dashed ellipses
show portions of the frontal cortices with right sulcal effacement. (b) Unenhanced CT detection of stroke:
the "insular ribbon sign," displayed using standard "window width" and "center level" gray scale settings.
Unenhanced CT at the level of the Sylvian fissure shows left insular hypodensity (white arrow), an
additional sign of infarction, the "insular ribbon sign," with loss of cortical/subcortical "gray–white"
differentiation and mild effacement of the Sylvian fissure and adjacent sulci by mass effect. (c)
Unenhanced CT detection of stroke: the "insular ribbon sign," shown with optimized "stroke window"
display parameters. Same image as Figure 2.2a, however now with optimized display parameters for the
detection of small changes in gray–white matter attenuation. Display parameters – with narrow window
width and center level settings (i.e. "stroke windows") – are optimized to exaggerate the subtle reduction in
attenuation accompanying acute cytotoxic and vasogenic edema.

(e.g. 30 HU width, 30 HU center level; Figure 2.2b,c) during image review [2]. Because gray matter is more vulnerable to ischemia and demonstrates 10–15 HU difference in density with white matter, ischemic hypoattenuation is best appreciated in gray matter structures, manifesting as defects in the basal ganglia or loss of gray–white matter differentiation in the cortical and insular ribbons.

EVIDENCE AT A GLANCE

Quantifying infarct burden using NCCT may be improved using the Alberta Stroke Program Early Computed Tomography Score (ASPECTS) [3]. It provides a semiquantitative estimation of infarct size and demonstrates good interobserver reliability. The improved reliability owes to its use of predominantly gray-matter structures to evaluate ischemic change. ASPECTS divides the middle cerebral artery (MCA) territory into ten regions: caudate, lentiform nucleus, posterior limb of the internal capsule (only purely white matter structure), insula, and six cortical regions (Figure 2.1B). For each region that demonstrates ischemic hypoattenuation, a single point is subtracted such that ten represents a normal scan and lower numbers indicate larger infarcts. While the original system utilized only two NCCT slices for evaluation, the current formulation requires inspection of all images to document ischemic changes. ASPECTS appears useful for predicting the clinical response to intra-arterial therapy (IAT).

Large vessel occlusions may be detected on NCCT as a hyperdense vessel segment (Figure 2.3). The previously reported sensitivity of this imaging finding is low (15–30%), which is related to overly thick (i.e. 5–10 mm) image reconstruction. Based on recent studies, hyperdense clots can be reliably identified (up to 90% of strokes) when images are reconstructed to 2.5 mm or thinner. Hyperdense clot lengths of 8 mm or greater appear to be resistant to IV tPA, as will be discussed later. More distal clots in the third-order branches may be identified as "dot" signs. Table 2.1 summarizes the advantages and disadvantages of NCCT.

Computed tomography angiography (CTA)

Neurovascular imaging is a critical diagnostic test for locating arterial occlusions and evaluating the

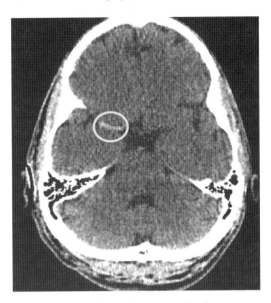

Figure 2.3 Unenhanced CT signs of early stroke – the "hyperdense middle cerebral artery (MCA)" sign. Hyperdensity is seen in the right middle cerebral artery (circle), consistent with and – in the setting of acute onset of stroke symptoms – highly specific for the presence of intraluminal occlusive clot.

underlying cause of stroke (e.g. large artery atherosclerosis). CT angiography is the best noninvasive method to evaluate the vessels of the head and neck, and demonstrates greater than 95% sensitivity and specificity for diagnosing proximal artery occlusion. It may be tailored to optimally visualize the arteries or the veins. CTA requires intravenous administration of a bolus of iodinated contrast solution (approximately 100 mL) via a power injector. The CT scanner is programmed to detect the arrival of the radiopaque contrast within the aortic arch, and then triggers scanning for optimal vascular opacification. With modern multidetector scanners, images of the head and neck arteries can be obtained in under 15 seconds, making this modality less prone to motion artifact.

The obvious downsides to CTA are radiation exposure and utilization of iodinated contrast, which may result in allergic reactions or glomerular injury in patients with diabetes or pre-existing renal impairment. The benefits however are high-resolution images from the aortic arch to the tertiary branches of the intracranial arteries. In fact, CTA is often used as an arbiter when there is discordance between

Table 2.1 Advantages/disadvantages of noncontrast computed tomography

Advantages/ pearls	Disadvantages/pitfalls
Widely available	Uses ionizing radiation
Minimal scan time (seconds)	Limited sensitivity and reliability for detecting early ischemic changes
Does not require complicated postprocessing	Imaging may be obscured by metallic streak artifact from surgical or endovascular implants
Accurate method for detecting intracranial hemorrhage	
Narrow window width settings improve ischemic lesion detection	
Thin section reconstruction allows for reliable identification of proximal artery occlusion	

carotid duplex imaging and magnetic resonance angiography for the degree of carotid stenosis. This advantage stems from the fact that CTA is resistant to flow-related changes unlike the other two tests. Similarly, CTA is the best noninvasive test for distinguishing total occlusion versus hairline residual lumen in cervical carotid disease. In this scenario, delayed imaging through the neck is valuable to detect slow antegrade flow. However, this lack of flow information on CTA limits evaluation of pathology such as arteriovenous malformations, where early artery-to-vein shunting cannot be detected on the static CTA images. An additional challenge to CTA is heavy arterial calcification, which can obscure the adjacent vessel lumen and impair evaluation of the degree of vessel stenosis.

Given the large axial imaging dataset, diagnosis of vessel abnormalities is facilitated by image postprocessing. In particular, maximum intensity projection (MIP) images (Figure 2.4a) of the intracranial circulation provide an easy way to detect proximal arterial occlusions that may be amenable to catheter-based therapy. These images depict the highest density along a particular imaging ray. For evaluation of the intracranial arteries, MIP images reformatted to 20–30 mm thickness with 3–5 mm overlap can be created in axial, coronal, and sagittal planes quickly at the scanner console. More complex postprocessing techniques include curved reformats, multiplanar volume reformats and volume rendered images. Curved reformats depict the entire course of a particular vessel in a single two-dimensional image, and provide a good evaluation

of arterial steno-occlusive disease in the neck, such as at the carotid bifurcation. The other techniques are less helpful for ischemic stroke evaluation, and are routinely used in aneurysm detection and treatment planning.

In addition to information regarding vessel patency, CTA source images (CTA-SI) provide a sensitive evaluation of ischemic changes within the brain parenchyma. Parenchymal hypoattenuation on CTA-SI represents decreased contrast opacification within the capillary bed, and is more readily detectable than NCCT hypodensity. Based on older literature, the size of the CTA-SI hypodense lesion has been taken as a good approximation of established core infarction (region of irreversible tissue injury).

> **⚠ CAUTION**
>
> Recent data from newer-generation scanners have shown that the volume of CTA-SI tissue hypodensity may significantly overestimate the core infarct and is strongly dependent on the timing of image acquisition after contrast injection [4]. Shorter time to imaging yields greater lesion sizes as there is less time for the contrast to traverse the pial collaterals and reach the capillary bed.

There have been numerous studies on the utility of CTA for grading of pial collateral strength. While

Axial

Coronal

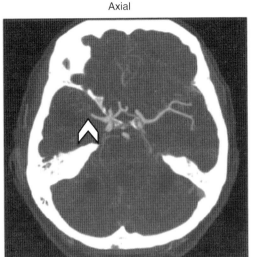

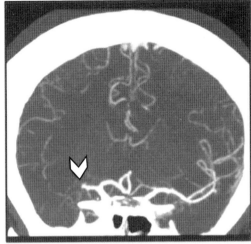

(a)

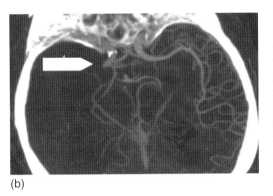

(b)

Figure 2.4 (a) Circle of Willis computed tomography angiography (CTA) for vascular assessment of acute embolic stroke. Axial and coronal CTA thick slab maximum intensity projection (MIP) images, showing a proximal right middle cerebral artery (MCA) occlusion (chevron). (b) Malignant collateral profile: head CTA MIP shows occlusion (thick arrow) of the origin of the right middle cerebral artery (MCA), with the absence of collateral vessels in the right inferior division of the MCA when compared to the left inferior division.

these studies have shown better outcomes with stronger collaterals, these grading schemes are not clinically useful for individual patient decision making as their specificity for clinical outcomes is often poor (i.e. outcomes are highly variable within collateral grades). However, a malignant CTA collateral pattern has been described recently, which is highly specific for a large infarct at presentation and may be useful for predicting a poor outcome despite treatment [5]. This malignant pattern is defined as the complete absence of vessels within a large cortical area of >50% of one MCA division (i.e. approximately 75 mL) (Figure 2.4b). With the emergence of volume CT scanning (e.g. 320-slice scanners), time-resolved angiography may allow for a better characterization of pial collaterals.

Table 2.2 summarizes the advantages and disadvantages of CTA.

Computed tomography perfusion (CTP)

CT perfusion is a dynamic contrast imaging method which seeks to characterize the degree of perfusion impairment within the ischemic tissue and thereby infer the viability of the brain parenchyma and risk of ischemic injury without reperfusion. The technique involves the administration of a bolus of contrast (approximately 35–50 mL at 7 mL/s) via a large-bore (18–20 gauge) intravenous line placed in the antecubital fossa. Scanning begins a few seconds after contrast injection, and involves rapid and repeated imaging of a fixed brain volume to record the first pass transit of contrast through

Table 2.2 Advantages/ disadvantages of computed tomography angiography (CTA)

Advantages/pearls	Disadvantages/pitfalls
Excellent noninvasive technique to obtain high-resolution imaging of vascular anatomy from the aortic arch to the intracranial vessels	Risks related to additional radiation exposure and iodinated contrast administration
Quick and does not require complex postprocessing for ischemic stroke evaluation	Provides a static image of cerebral vasculature (i.e. no flow information)
CTA source images provide a more sensitive evaluation of parenchymal ischemic change than noncontrast computed tomography	Heavy calcification or metallic implant limits evaluation of vessel patency
	CTA source images do not provide reliable information on brain tissue viability

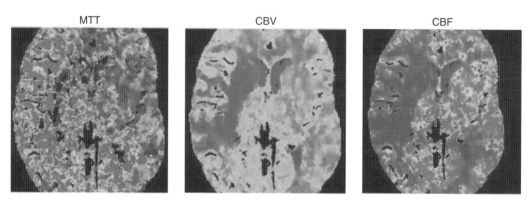

Figure 2.5 CT perfusion maps. Axial computed tomography perfusion (CTP) images in the territory of an acute right MCA occlusion on CTA. The mean transit time (MTT, measured in seconds) is elevated (red pixels), with a concomitant decrease in both cerebral blood volume (CBV, measured in mL/100 g brain, dark blue pixels) and cerebral blood flow (CBF, measured in mL/100 g/min, dark blue pixels), consistent with severe hypoperfusion, and suggesting ischemia. The CT-CBV and CT-CBF deficits are "matched," indicating no additional "at-risk" penumbral tissue surrounding the critically ischemic region. (See also Plate 2.5)

the ischemic bed. This cine imaging should be carried out for at least 60–75 seconds to prevent truncation of the concentration–time curve, which will lead to underestimation of cerebral blood volume. There are numerous methods to derive tissue-level perfusion parameters, which may be broadly classified as deconvolution and nondeconvolution based. Deconvolution corrects for bolus delay and dispersion up to the level of a user-defined or automatically selected arterial input function, which is often placed at the proximal arteries. Some of the commonly used parameters are described below (Figure 2.5).

Mean transit time (MTT): MTT is the average time taken by a tracer to pass through a tissue. With respect to the cerebral vasculature, it is the average time taken for blood from entering at the arterial input to leaving at the venous output of the vascular network.

Time to peak (TTP) and Tmax: TTP is a nondeconvolution based metric which is defined as the time lag between first arrival of the contrast agent within major arterial vessels included in the section and the local bolus peak in the brain tissue. Tmax is a similar parameter derived from deconvolution analysis, and represents the time at which the tissue residue function reaches maximum intensity.

Cerebral blood volume (CBV): CBV is defined as the volume occupied by blood in a region of interest. This is usually expressed as milliliters per 100 grams of tissue.

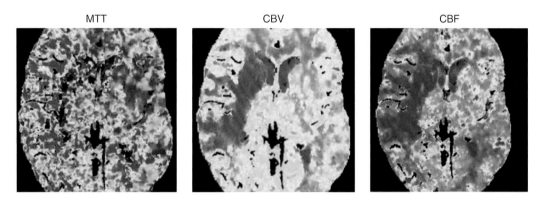

MTT   CBV   CBF

Plate 2.5 CT perfusion maps. Axial computed tomography perfusion (CTP) images in the territory of an acute right MCA occlusion on CTA. The mean transit time (MTT, measured in seconds) is elevated (red pixels), with a concomitant decrease in both cerebral blood volume (CBV, measured in mL/100 g brain, dark blue pixels) and cerebral blood flow (CBF, measured in mL/100 g/min, dark blue pixels), consistent with severe hypoperfusion, and suggesting ischemia. The CT-CBV and CT-CBF deficits are "matched," indicating no additional "at-risk" penumbral tissue surrounding the critically ischemic region.

Stroke, First Edition. Edited by Kevin M. Barrett and James F. Meschia.
© 2013 John Wiley & Sons, Ltd. Published 2013 by John Wiley & Sons, Ltd.

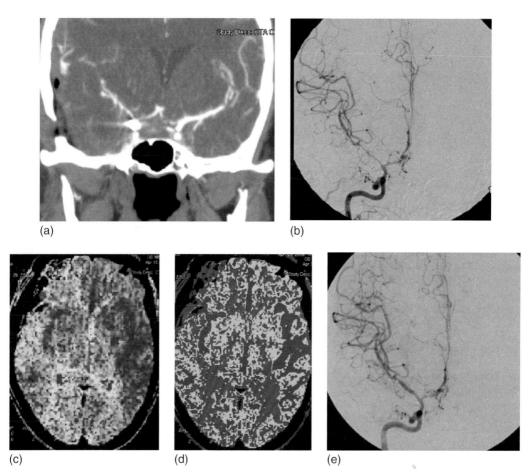

(a) (b)

(c) (d) (e)

Plate 5.9 CT and catheter angiogram images (a,b) demonstrating right middle cerebral artery (MCA) vasospasm 6 days after a ruptured right posterior communicating artery aneurysm. The CT perfusion images (c,d) show increased mean transit time (c) and reduced blood flow (d) in the right MCA vascular territory. Vasospasm was treated with balloon angioplasty (e).

Table 2.3 Advantages/disadvantages of computed tomography perfusion (CTP)

Advantages/pearls	Disadvantages/pitfalls
Provides a sensitive evaluation of altered brain hemodynamics, and can be used to rule out ischemic pathologies	Patient risk related to additional radiation exposure and contrast administration
When MRI is not readily available, CTP may be the best alternative to obtain hemodynamic information	CTP is not validated for thrombolysis decision making, and suffers from poor standardization of image acquisition, postprocessing algorithms, and analytic methods
	Uncertainty whether quantification of perfusion parameters is robust enough for threshold-based approaches to tissue characterization
	Highly sensitive to patient motion

Cerebral blood flow (CBF): CBF is defined as the flow through a given region of interest and is expressed in milliliters of blood per 100 grams of brain tissue per minute.

CBF, CBV, and MTT are related by the central volume theorem: CBF = CBV/MTT, which demonstrates that cerebral blood flow increases with an increase in cerebral blood volume and falls with an increase in the mean transit time.

Currently, CTP images acquired from the scanner are sent to a stand-alone workstation for processing. Various vendors provide software packages that use the above processing algorithms to convert the raw images into visual perfusion maps. Modern multidetector CT scanners have allowed for greater z-axis (superior–inferior) coverage, with whole-brain perfusion imaging now possible with the newest-generation scanners.

Until recently, the core infarct has been defined as the region of low cerebral blood volume on CTP maps with varying thresholds reported in the literature. However, more recent data support the use of thresholded CBF for delineation of irreversible injury [6]. The penumbral region (at risk for infarction without reperfusion) has been variably defined using abnormally low CBF or prolonged MTT. Clearly, CT perfusion requires better validation before it can be used for treatment decision making. The primary challenge is the lack of standardization of postprocessing algorithms and thresholds for defining infarcted versus threatened tissue [7]. These thresholds vary depending on the specific CTP software used. Another challenge is whether perfusion imaging is truly quantifiable. Numerous studies have demonstrated significant errors in perfusion

measurement, which would make threshold approaches invalid. Table 2.3 summarizes the advantages and disadvantages of CTP.

> ★ **TIPS AND TRICKS**
>
> Pending further evidence, perfusion imaging should be reserved only for assessing whether or not an ischemic syndrome is present given its high sensitivity to alterations in brain hemodynamics. A stroke is ruled out if the hemodynamic parameters are entirely normal. To date, perfusion imaging has no demonstrated utility for deciding whether a patient should receive reperfusion therapy.

Diffusion-weighted imaging (DWI)

The advent of MRI ushered in a new era in neuro-imaging. Its major advantage over CT for acute ischemic stroke evaluation is diffusion-weighted imaging. DWI became clinically available in the 1990s and remains the most accurate method for detecting hyperacute infarction.

> ⚙ **SCIENCE REVISITED**
>
> While the technical aspects of this imaging technique are beyond the scope of this chapter, DWI is designed to measure the diffusion of water molecules within the brain tissue, and is particularly useful in an acute ischemic stroke where the diffusion of water molecules is restricted.

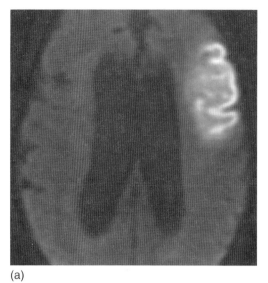
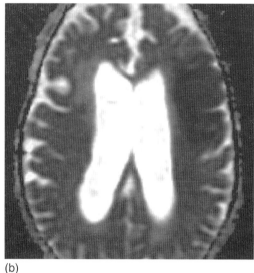

(a)   (b)

Figure 2.6 MR diffusion-weighted imaging (DWI) in acute ischemic stroke. (a) DWI imaging sequence depicting high signal in the left frontal lobe, with corresponding low signal ("restricted diffusion") on the "apparent diffusion coefficient" (ADC) map (b). These findings are highly sensitive and specific for the detection of acute infarct "core" – tissue likely to be irreversibly infarcted despite early, robust reperfusion.

Ultrafast echo planar imaging techniques are utilized to minimize patient motion artifact, and result in a total imaging time of approximately 2 minutes.

Multiple diffusion imaging sequences are produced clinically: isotropic DWI, apparent diffusion coefficient (ADC), and exponential maps. Clinical interpretation requires evaluation of the DWI and ADC maps in conjunction because of the issue of "T2 shine through." Restricted diffusion appears hyperintense (i.e. bright) on the isotropic DWI sequence (Figure 2.6). However, there is also T2 signal information on these images, such that hyperintensity owing to T2 effects may be misinterpreted as restricted diffusion. The ADC images isolate the changes related to true diffusion restriction, which appear as hypointense (i.e. dark) signal. Therefore, areas of acute infarction appear bright on DWI and dark on ADC. Parenthetically, the exponential images are similar to DWI but do not have T2 information (i.e. bright signal equates to restricted diffusion). However, the exponential sequence is less commonly used because the image contrast is less than that for DWI, which may affect reader sensitivity. The sensitivity and specificity of DWI for detecting infarction in the first 6 hours is above 90%.

One issue that has raised doubts regarding the clinical utility of DWI is potential reversibility of diffusion restriction. However, numerous recent studies have demonstrated that this phenomenon is rare, involves minimal volumes of tissue (approximately 3 mL median volume) and does not alter clinical outcomes. Improved outcomes that have been reported in cases with diffusion restriction are likely related to accompanying penumbral salvage, as reperfusion is a sine qua non of this phenomenon. Based on the best available evidence, numerous expert panels have given DWI a class I (level of evidence A) recommendation for core infarct imaging.

Due to its high accuracy for depicting very early infarction, DWI may reveal distinct patterns of ischemia, including lacunar, embolic, and watershed patterns, which can provide important clues regarding the etiology of the stroke. Moreover, in patients with transient ischemic attack, DWI evidence of infarction has been shown to predict a higher risk of early stroke, and should prompt more urgent diagnostic workup. Table 2.4 summarizes the advantages and disadvantages of DWI.

Gradient echo (GRE) T2*-weighted imaging

GRE T2*-weighted imaging is highly sensitive to blood breakdown products due to their paramagnetic properties, which result in signal loss and thus

Table 2.4 Advantages/disadvantages of MRI diffusion-weighted imaging

Advantages/pearls	Disadvantages/pitfalls
Most accurate method for delineating irreversible tissue injury (core infarct)	Contraindicated in people with pacemakers or other ferromagnetic implants
Rapid imaging time	Not as widely available as CT in the community setting, but is readily available in academic and comprehensive stroke centers where intra-arterial stroke therapy is offered
Predicts early stroke risk in patients with transient ischemic attack	
Does not use ionizing radiation	
Does not require use of a contrast agent	

Table 2.5 Advantages/disadvantages of MR angiography

Advantages/pearls	Disadvantages/pitfalls
Accurate for diagnosing proximal artery occlusions amenable to intra-arterial therapy	May overestimate vessel stenosis due to flow artifact
May be performed without contrast administration	Susceptible to patient motion artifact

appear dark. Studies have shown that $T2^*$-weighted imaging is as accurate as NCCT for detecting acute intracranial hemorrhage, and is superior for chronic bleeds. More recently, susceptibility weighted imaging has emerged as an extension of $T2^*$-weighted imaging. It provides phase and magnitude information from high-resolution three-dimensional GRE-based sequences that can accentuate differences in magnetic susceptibility.

Magnetic resonance angiography (MRA)

MR angiography is a common vascular imaging test, and may be performed either with noncontrast or contrast-enhanced techniques. The imaging resolution is inferior to CTA, and the images are susceptible to flow-related artifact (particularly without contrast). Noncontrast MRA utilizes time-of-flight (TOF) techniques, and relies on signals generated by flowing blood. However, such techniques may result in overestimation of stenosis severity and length due to turbulent flow. This is minimized with gadolinium-enhanced imaging. Three-dimensional TOF technique is typically performed for the intracranial circulation, while gadolinium is used for imaging the aortic arch and neck vessels. For the question of proximal intracranial artery occlusion, three-dimensional TOF MRA performs reasonably well with approximately 85% sensitivity and 90% specificity. Table 2.5 summarizes the advantages and disadvantages of MRA.

Magnetic resonance perfusion weighted imaging (MRP)

The principles of MRI perfusion imaging are similar to CTP. Dynamic brain imaging is performed after the injection of gadolinium to measure the first-pass transit of contrast through the cerebral vasculature. Postprocessing techniques yield similar perfusion parameters to CTP, which have been previously described. Renal function should be tested prior to gadolinium administration, as gadolinium carries the risk of nephrogenic systemic fibrosis (NSF) in patients with severe renal impairment. NSF results in fibrosis of the skin and internal organs and may be fatal. Physicians should refer to their local institutional policy on gadolinium administration for further guidance. More recently, perfusion imaging using arterial spin labeling has been introduced into clinical practice, and does not require the administration of a contrast agent. Instead, endogenous contrast is created by tagging arterial water spins prior to entry into the brain. Similar to CTP, MRI perfusion imaging demonstrates significant errors in cerebral perfusion quantification, for both dynamic contrast methods and arterial spin labeling. Therefore, MRP cannot be used to characterize at-risk tissue and is not validated for decision making regarding thrombolysis. It should be used only to assess if the patient's symptoms are ischemic in origin. Table 2.6 summarizes the advantages and disadvantages of MRP.

Table 2.6 Advantages/disadvantages of MRI perfusion weighted imaging (MRP)

Advantages/pearls	Disadvantages/pitfalls
Does not use ionizing radiation	Contraindicated in people with pacemakers or other ferromagnetic implants
Provides a sensitive evaluation for altered cerebral hemodynamics	Gadolinium carries the risk of nephrogenic systemic fibrosis in patients with severe renal impairment
	MRP is not validated for thrombolysis decision making
	Uncertainty whether quantification of perfusion parameters is robust enough for threshold-based approaches to tissue characterization

Clinical considerations

The value of any test is measured by whether it provides information that is relevant to patient management. As such, the imaging approach is highly dependent on the clinical setting. The following discussion is broadly divided into ischemic and hemorrhagic disease.

Imaging evaluation of acute cerebral ischemia

Imaging workup for intravenous tissue type plasminogen activator (IV tPA)

The only imaging finding that is an absolute contraindication to IV tPA is the presence of acute intracranial hemorrhage. This is best evaluated using noncontrast head CT scan. However, numerous studies have shown that MRI with T2*-weighted imaging is equally accurate for identifying acute intracranial hemorrhage [8], and thus MRI may be performed in centers where this modality is readily available. It should be noted that MRI T2*-weighted imaging is highly sensitive to chronic microbleeds (<5 mm area of signal loss without surrounding edema).

EVIDENCE AT A GLANCE

In a study of 570 patients treated with IV tPA within 6 hours, there was a small but not statistically significant increase in the risk of symptomatic hemorrhage in patients with chronic microbleeds (5.8% vs. 2.7%) [9]. Based on this study, the benefit of IV tPA should not be withheld from patients harboring such findings. It remains uncertain whether there is a higher risk of thrombolysis among patients with more numerous microbleeds (e.g. >5).

Importantly, the presence of extensive ischemic changes (i.e. involving greater than one-third of the MCA territory) on NCCT is only a relative contraindication to IV tPA within the 3-hour window, as there are conflicting data on whether such findings preclude treatment benefit [10]. Similarly, quantifying infarct burden using the Alberta Stroke Program Early CT Score (ASPECTS) on NCCT does not predict treatment response to IV tPA. However, in the 3 to 4.5-hour window, major ischemic changes are an absolute contraindication because such changes were an ECASS III exclusion criterion [11]. In this trial, pretreatment imaging was mostly performed with NCCT although MRI was performed in some centers.

★ TIPS AND TRICKS

Given the strong time dependence of IV tPA benefit, a clear emphasis should be placed on rapid imaging acquisition and interpretation. Guidelines recommend that brain imaging be performed within 25 minutes of the patient's arrival and that interpretation be completed by 45 minutes, such that IV tPA can be administered within 1 hour of arrival.

As previously discussed, NCCT findings such as parenchymal hypoattenuation, loss of gray–white matter distinction, and cortical swelling confirm the diagnosis of acute ischemic stroke. Of these parenchymal changes, hypoattenuation of the gray matter structures, including the basal ganglia, insula, and cortical ribbon, is the most easily discernible. In addition, the clot may be visualized as a hyperdense vessel or dot (when involving smaller distal vessels) sign. Imaging may reveal other etiologies for the patient's symptoms which would preclude treatment, including a tumor or abscess with surrounding vasogenic edema or posterior reversible encephalopathy syndrome.

Recent data suggest that imaging may be used to identify patients who may be less likely to benefit from IV tPA. In particular, proximal artery occlusion on vessel imaging has been shown to have a relatively low rate of early recanalization with intravenous thrombolysis (approximately 5% for ICA terminus and 30% for proximal MCA), and may benefit from additional catheter-based treatment. Additionally, clot lengths of ≥8 mm determined using thin-section (≤2.5 mm) NCCT have been shown to have a very low probability (<5%) of IV tPA-induced recanalization [12].

> ### ☝ CAUTION
>
> Proximal arterial occlusion and clot length >8 mm should not preclude IV tPA treatment as some patients may still benefit. Their presence should prompt consideration of rapid triage to interventional therapy in appropriate patients.

> ### CLINICAL PEARLS
>
> - Exclusion of intracranial hemorrhage is the only imaging finding required before the administration of IV tPA for eligible patients.
> - Imaging must be performed and interpreted in a rapid fashion.
> - Imaging evidence of significant clot burden may predict poor response to IV tPA, and supports early activation of the endovascular stroke team.

Imaging workup for intra-arterial stroke therapy

After the exclusion of intracranial hemorrhage, patients should then undergo more advanced imaging to evaluate their eligibility for intra-arterial therapy. Vessel imaging is a critical first step to identify proximal occlusions amenable to IAT, and can obviate unnecessary catheter angiography in patients whose major arteries are patent.

> ### ☆ TIPS AND TRICKS
>
> Neurovascular imaging should not delay IV tPA administration in eligible patients. If two large-bore intravenous catheters are available, then tPA can be administered via one of them, while the other is used to inject the contrast agent necessary to obtain the CTA.

For proximal occlusions, IAT yields significantly higher rates of reperfusion (70–90% TIMI/TICI 2–3) compared to IV tPA. Moreover, vessel imaging often provides important information to the neuro-interventionalist for treatment planning. Knowledge of the anatomy of the aortic arch and cervical vessels, including presence of marked tortuosity or significant steno-occlusive disease, may impact the choice of vascular access catheters and whether angioplasty and stenting of cervical stenosis will be required. In older patients, atherosclerotic disease at the carotid bifurcation is a common cause of embolic stroke, while arterial dissection is more prevalent in younger patients.

There are relatively few data concerning parenchymal imaging findings that predict the clinical response to IAT. As such, there is no consensus regarding the optimal parenchymal imaging approach. PROACT II, the only formal trial to demonstrate the clinical efficacy of IAT, utilized noncontrast CT evidence of a large infarct (greater than one-third MCA territory or significant mass effect with midline shift) as its only imaging exclusion criteria in addition to the presence of hemorrhage. However, limitations of this approach include poor sensitivity and limited interobserver agreement.

Therefore, advanced imaging selection for IAT is increasingly being used. Emerging evidence points to the important role of core infarct size in determining outcomes after IAT [13]. This has been shown using various modalities, including Xenon CT, MRI DWI, CT perfusion, and NCCT. Of these techniques, the most accurate and reliable is MRI diffusion imaging. It has the added advantage of allowing straightforward infarct volume quantification. Based on available data, acute DWI lesion volumes greater than 70–100 mL are highly predictive of poor outcomes despite successful IAT. In the clinical setting, infarct volume is typically calculated manually using the ABC/2 method (i.e. ellipsoid approximation) but future automated algorithms may provide a more precise measure.

While some point to the reduced availability of MRI in the treatment setting, this is unlikely to be true at comprehensive stroke centers that offer IAT. Importantly, the clinical utility of perfusion imaging to assess the size of viable but hypoperfused tissue appears limited given that patients with proximal occlusions who have a small core infarct are almost assured to have a significant volume of penumbral tissue. Instead, utilizing the NIH Stroke Scale (NIHSS) to document a significant neurologic deficit is more informative for suggesting the presence of a clinically significant penumbra, which can then be defined as the combination of a proximal occlusion, small core infarct (e.g. <70–100 mL) and significant deficit (e.g. NIHSS score >8–10) [14].

If MRI is unavailable or contraindicated (e.g. ferromagnetic implants), evidence supports using NCCT parenchymal evaluation based on ASPECTS (Figure 2.1b). This semiquantitative method for infarct size determination partitions the MCA territory into ten distinct regions. When hypoattenuation is identified in a region, a point is subtracted such that lower scores indicate larger infarcts. Using ASPECTS, a post hoc analysis of PROACT II demonstrated that patients with NCCT ASPECTS >7 demonstrated a treatment benefit while those with ASPECTS 0–7 had no better outcomes with IAT [15]. However, more recent data from studies of the Penumbra Stroke System suggest that patients with ASPECTS 5–7 may benefit from early revascularization, and that only scores between 0 and 4 should be excluded. Clearly, prospective validation of these thresholds is needed. While some centers utilize CT perfusion to delineate the core infarct size, this remains poorly validated as discussed above. Challenges to CTP include poor standardization of acquisition and analysis and questionable reliability of perfusion quantification. The imaging approach to acute ischemic stroke at Massachusetts General Hospital is provided in Figure 2.7.

CLINICAL PEARLS

- Vessel imaging with CTA or MRA can rapidly and accurately identify proximal intracranial artery occlusions amenable to IAT.
- Pretreatment core infarct volume predicts the clinical response to IAT.
- A clinically significant penumbra for IAT decision making may be defined as a proximal occlusion, small core infarct, and significant neurologic deficit.

Imaging evaluation of acute nontraumatic intracranial hemorrhage

Approximately 10 to 15% of all strokes are hemorrhagic. Acute hemorrhage is most easily identified on NCCT, where it appears hyperdense (60–80 HU) to brain parenchyma. On MRI, hemorrhage has a variable appearance depending on the age and breakdown products of the blood (Table 2.7).

The imaging workup of nontraumatic intracranial hemorrhage seeks to identify treatable vascular etiologies. The most common causes include cerebral aneurysms and pial or dural arteriovenous malformations (AVMs). The location of the hemorrhage (extra- versus intraparenchymal) provides clues to the likely cause, and will influence the subsequent imaging workup.

Subarachnoid hemorrhage (SAH): acute SAH is best identified on NCCT as hyperdensity in the CSF spaces surrounding the brain (Figure 2.8), and may often be seen layering in the ventricles when there is intraventricular extension. On MRI, SAH may be identified using fluid attenuated inversion recovery (FLAIR) imaging, where it appears as hyperintense signal within the CSF spaces (which are normally dark). The primary cause of nontraumatic or spontaneous SAH is a ruptured cerebral aneurysm. Other vascular causes include intracranial dissection, vasculitis, mycotic aneurysm, dural AVM, and cervical fistulas. For diagnostic purposes, spontaneous SAH may be divided into perimesencephalic or diffuse patterns. This distinction has important bearing on the yield of the aneurysm workup, as well as the clinical course. A perimesencephalic pattern accounts for approximately 10% of SAH cases, is centered anterior to the brainstem, and can extend to involve the ambient and suprasellar cisterns. There can be involvement of the proximal anterior interhemispheric and proximal sylvian cisterns, but the remainder of these cisterns should not be filled with blood and there should be no intraventricular extension. Patients with this SAH pattern are highly unlikely to have an intracranial aneurysm (~5%), and in the vast majority of cases have an excellent clinical course.

Noninvasive vascular imaging has become the first-line test for aneurysm detection and treatment planning. With its high spatial resolution, CTA has excellent accuracy for identifying aneurysms.

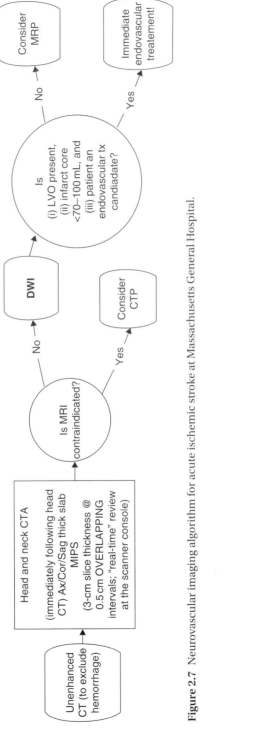

Figure 2.7 Neurovascular imaging algorithm for acute ischemic stroke at Massachusetts General Hospital.

Table 2.7 Serial stages of hemorrhage appearance on MRI

Stage	Biochemistry	T1	T2	T2* Susceptibility (strongly paramagnetic)	Time
Hyperacute	Oxyhemoglobin/serum	↓	↑		minutes–hours
Acute	Deoxyhemoglobin	←→	↓	↓↓	hours–days
Subacute, early	Intracellular methemoglobin	↑	←→	↓	days–weeks
Subacute, late	Extracellular methemoglobin	↑	↑		weeks–months
Chronic	Hemosiderin	↓	↓	↓↓	months–years

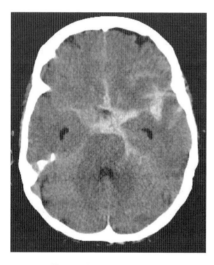

Figure 2.8 Diffuse subarachnoid hemorrhage. An axial section of an unenhanced head CT scan demonstrates hyperdensity, consistent with acute subarachnoid hemorrhage, in the basal cisterns and sulci, which typically contain hypodense cerebrospinal fluid. The distribution of the hemorrhage suggests a possible aneurysm of the left middle cerebral artery as a source.

A large comparative study of 64-detector CTA against gold standard digital subtraction angiography (DSA) revealed 100% sensitivity and specificity for aneurysms sized 3 mm or greater [16]. However, the sensitivity for tiny aneurysms (<3 mm) is lower with variable rates reported in the literature (70–95%). Several authors have recommended that a negative CTA in the setting of perimesencephalic SAH is sufficient and obviates the need for DSA [17]. In contrast, in patients with a diffuse SAH pattern, DSA is warranted even if initial CTA is negative, and a second DSA at 5–7 days should be strongly considered if the first DSA is negative as the yield for aneurysm detection may be as high as 15% in this setting. Finally, if the SAH is predominantly in a peripheral sulcal distribution, there should be a high clinical suspicion for vasculitis or mycotic aneurysm.

For proximal aneurysms arising from or near the circle of Willis, CTA provides suitable anatomic information for treatment planning in the majority of cases. Important information for deciding between surgical clipping and endovascular coiling include aneurysm size and location, dome-to-neck ratio, location of adjacent branch vessels and presence of intra-aneurysmal thrombus. Post-processed images such as multiplanar reformats and volume rendered images are often helpful for depicting these aneurysm characteristics. Imaging assessment and notification of findings to the neurovascular team should be performed urgently as early aneurysm closure (e.g. within 24 hours) is associated with more favorable outcomes.

Intraparenchymal hemorrhage (IPH): approximately 85% of IPHs are primary (i.e. no causative anatomic lesion) and most often associated with hypertension. Hypertensive bleeds typically affect the basal ganglia, pons, and deep cerebellar nuclei. Imaging is critical for identifying potential causes of secondary IPH, which include AVM, aneurysm, venous sinus thrombosis, tumor, and vasculitis. Vascular lesions have a high risk of recurrent hemorrhage, and should be treated when discovered. Young (<45 years) normotensive patients with IPH have a particularly high incidence (50–65%) of underlying vascular abnormality, the majority of which are AVMs and aneurysms [18].

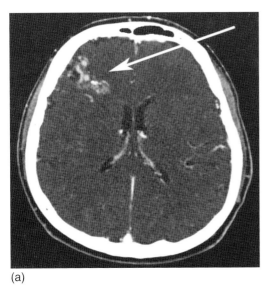
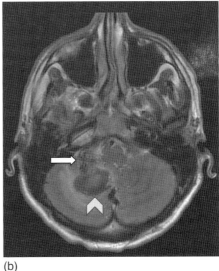

(a) (b)

Figure 2.9 (a) CTA appearance of arteriovenous malformation. There are numerous enhancing vessels in the right frontal lobe consistent with a brain arteriovenous malformation (arrow). Note the compact AVM nidus of tiny vessels medially and the enlarged draining vein laterally. (b) MRI appearance of hemorrhagic arteriovenous malformation. An axial section of a T2-weighted MRI demonstrating a right inferior cerebellar arteriovenous malformation (flow voids, arrow), with an associated right cerebellar parenchymal hematoma (chevron; see Table 2.7 for details of the signal intensity changes with time post hemorrhage).

On CTA, anatomic clues to the diagnosis of AVM include numerous and enlarged vessels corresponding to feeding arteries, the vascular nidus or draining veins as well as associated calcifications (Figure 2.9a). Similar findings may be seen on MRI, where the abnormal vessels appear as flow voids on T2-weighted imaging (Figure 2.9b). However, small AVMs may be easily overlooked on anatomic imaging. Unlike CTA images which are static, MRA techniques offer a noninvasive means of imaging arteriovenous shunting, and thus is a complementary diagnostic test for the noninvasive evaluation of brain AVMs and dural fistulas. Specifically, three-dimensional TOF MRA may reveal arterial flow-related enhancement within venous structures in such lesions. Flow dynamics may also be depicted using time-resolved MRI or CT angiography, but these techniques are more technically demanding.

Dural sinus or cortical vein thrombosis is a less common cause of IPH, but should always be considered, particularly in young to middle aged females who are postpartum or on oral contraceptives.

Intracranial veins are often opacified on CTA, and, if so, should be evaluated for filling defects or occlusion. Important mimics within the dural sinuses include arachnoid granulations, which are often seen on CTA as lobulated filling defects in the lateral aspects of the transverse sinuses, as well as hypoplasia of a transverse sinus. Suspected thrombosis should be confirmed on noncontrast CT as hyperdense clot within the vein or sinus. Dedicated CT or MR venography may be performed. Gradient echo imaging is often helpful for cortical vein thrombosis which appears as a serpentine area of signal loss (blooming artifact). DWI may reveal restricted diffusion (cytotoxic edema), elevated diffusion (vasogenic edema from venous congestion), or both.

Vasculopathy or mycotic aneurysm is another uncommon cause of IPH. These entities typically involve the medium and small vessels, and should be considered when parenchymal hemorrhage is seen in combination with peripheral subarachnoid hemorrhage and scattered focal infarcts. Vasculitic changes include beaded irregularity and

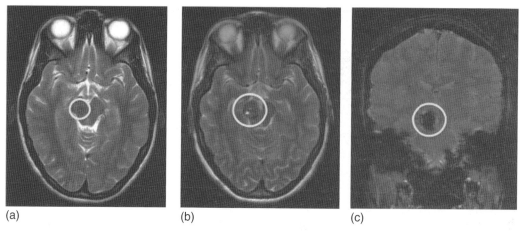

(a)   (b)   (c)

Figure 2.10 Typical MRI appearance of hemorrhagic cavernous malformation. (a) Right midbrain cavernous malformation (also known as a "cavernoma"), which was initially asymptomatic, seen as a small T2-weighted hyperintense lesion with a surrounding rim of hypointense signal (the so-called "popcorn" appearance). (b) Several months after the initial MRI, the patient presented with left-sided weakness and ataxia; T2-weighted MRI revealed a similar but larger lesion, suggesting new hemorrhage in the interval. (c) Coronal gradient-echo MRI sequence ("susceptibility imaging") showed a signal void "blooming artifact," typical of deoxyhemoglobin and hemosiderin blood breakdown products (see also Figure 2.8).

narrowing, which may be difficult to detect in smaller vessels on CTA. Collapsed MIP images are often helpful to evaluate these vessels, and may also help to detect distal saccular outpouchings consistent with mycotic aneurysms, which are often seen in the distal MCA branches given their higher flow. Also, MRI may suggest the diagnosis by revealing associated infarcts on DWI. Moreover, gradient echo images may help to detect mycotic aneurysms, which often appear as focal areas of signal loss.

In addition to three-dimensional TOF MRA, routine MRI is important for identifying other causes of IPH that would obviate the need for further vascular imaging. DWI may reveal restricted diffusion to suggest hemorrhagic transformation of an ischemic stroke. Hemorrhagic tumors such as metastases may be evident on postgadolinium imaging as multiple abnormally enhancing lesions. Cavernous malformations have a classic appearance on T2-weighted images as a focal area of central T2 bright signal surrounded by a dark rim of hemosiderin (Figure 2.10). Amyloid angiopathy results in numerous small foci of dark signal (microbleeds) distributed throughout the brain on gradient echo or susceptibility-weighted imaging.

The accuracy of CTA for identifying a vascular cause of IPH is high with sensitivity and specificity greater than 95% [18, 19]. Nonetheless, small lesions such as AVMs can be obscured by associated mass effect from the hematoma, and therefore DSA should be strongly considered in the setting of a negative CTA (and negative MRI if obtained). Deciding which patients should go on to DSA after a negative CTA is a matter of debate. In older patients (>45 years) with a history of hypertension who present with IPH in the basal ganglia or thalamus, the yield of DSA for identifying an underlying vascular abnormality has been reported to be exceedingly low [20]. While the posterior fossa is another common location for hypertensive bleeds, one study could not identify an independent predictor of underlying vascular lesion among 68 patients with posterior fossa IPH [19], suggesting that DSA should be performed in this setting when CTA is negative. In all other patients, DSA is the appropriate next step in evaluation. If the DSA is negative, repeat angiography should be considered after the resolution of the hematoma and associated mass effect (e.g. after 2–4 weeks).

In cases of primary IPH (i.e. no cause is identified), imaging may be helpful for prognostication and to

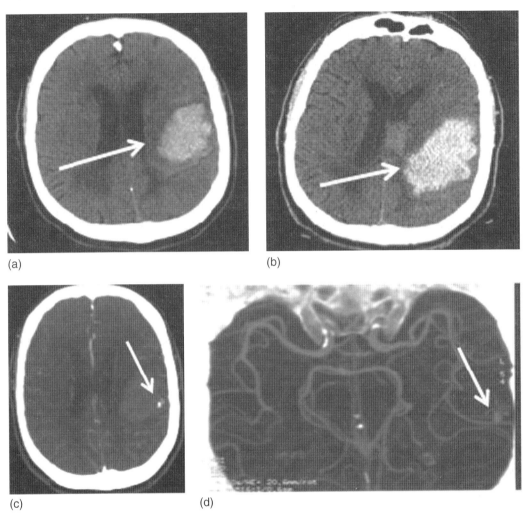

(a)

(b)

(c)

(d)

Figure 2.11 Computed tomography angiography (CTA) "spot sign". (a) Admission unenhanced head CT shows a large hyperdense left frontal hematoma (arrow). (b) On follow-up, 2–3 hours later, the hematoma had expanded (arrow). (c) Admission CT angiography (CTA) source images revealed a small focus of contrast extravasation, the "spot sign" (arrow). (d) The collapsed maximum intensity projection (MIP) CTA axial image at the circle of Willis level confirmed the presence of a high-density "spot sign" (arrow).

identify patients at high risk for hematoma expansion. In addition to a poor clinical exam at presentation (e.g. Glasgow Coma Scale score <9), imaging findings that are highly predictive of mortality and poor outcomes include a large hematoma volume (e.g. >60 mL) and the presence of intraventricular hemorrhage. Approximately one-third of patients found to have IPH within 3 to 6 hours of onset demonstrate further significant (>33% or 6 mL) hematoma growth, which is another independent predictor of worse outcomes. While treatments to prevent hematoma expansion require further clinical validation, identifying high-risk populations for hematoma growth may provide important prognostic information, guide decisions regarding early surgery, and allow more targeted patient selection in future trials of hemostatic therapy. Recent studies have supported the ability of CTA to predict hematoma growth by revealing contrast extravasation within the hemorrhage (the spot sign; Figure 2.11).

There are various working definitions of the spot sign. In general, a spot must be within the hematoma, demonstrate density much higher than the surrounding blood (e.g. ≥120 HU), and be discontinuous from vessels. It can take any morphology, and more than one may be identified within the hematoma. Recommended viewing settings are window width 200 HU and level 110 HU. Spot sign mimics include areas of focal calcification (which can be identified on the NCCT images) and enhancement within the choroid plexus for bleeds adjacent to the ventricles or with associated intraventricular blood. Additional spot sign characteristics that may further stratify rebleeding risk include the presence of three or more spots, maximum diameter of the largest spot ≥5 mm, and maximum attenuation of the largest spot ≥180 HU. These findings have been incorporated into a spot sign score (Table 2.8) [21], which has been demonstrated to independently predict significant hematoma growth, higher in-hospital mortality, and poor outcomes among survivors.

Table 2.8 Computed tomography angiography (CTA) "spot sign" score for predicting risk of hematoma expansion

Spot sign finding	Points
Number of spot signs	
1–2	1
≥3	2
Maximal axial length	
1–4 mm	0
≥5 mm	1
Maximum density (in Hounsfield Units, HU)	
120–179 HU	0
≥180 HU	1
Spot sign score	**Risk of bleed growth**
0	2%
1	33%
2	50%
3	94%
4	100%

The "spot sign" score is the sum of the individual components listed above; when multiple "spots" are present, the maximal measurements are obtained from the largest one. Note also that the recommended HU cutoff values for density are based on the specific CTA acquisition protocol used in the paper by Delgado Almandoz et al. [21], and may not be generalizable to other CTA protocols using different contrast agents, injection rates, and timing of imaging.

CLINICAL PEARLS

- Vascular imaging is critical to identify treatable causes of spontaneous intracranial hemorrhage.
- CTA is highly accurate for identifying aneurysms and arteriovenous malformations and is a first-line test for both diagnosis and treatment planning.
- Catheter angiography should be performed in most cases when noninvasive imaging does not reveal a source of hemorrhage.
- MRA with time-of-flight technique may allow detection of arteriovenous shunting and may be a complementary test.
- Contrast extravasation on CTA is a strong predictor of early and significant hematoma growth.

Conclusion

Neuroimaging is critical to the appropriate management of the acute stroke patient. The most important question is whether the stroke is ischemic or hemorrhagic in nature, as this will influence the diagnostic and therapeutic pathway. For ischemic strokes, IV tPA should be administered as rapidly as possible to eligible patients without evidence of intracranial hemorrhage. Further information should then be obtained regarding vessel status and the extent of the irreversibly injured brain to decide whether an endovascular approach is indicated. For hemorrhagic strokes, the location of the blood determines whether a vascular cause is likely and what type of vascular lesion is present. Noninvasive vessel imaging is highly accurate for diagnosing aneurysms and arteriovenous malformations, which are amenable to surgical or endovascular treatment approaches. Moreover, in primary intraparenchymal bleeds, imaging may predict the risk of early hematoma growth and offer a target for future hemostatic therapies. Ongoing research should bring many new and important insights in the near future.

Selected bibliography

1. Yoo AJ, Pulli B, Gonzalez RG. Imaging-based treatment selection for intravenous and intra-arterial stroke therapies: a comprehensive review. *Expert Rev Cardiovasc Ther* 2011; **9**: 857–76.

2. Lev MH, Farkas J, Gemmete JJ, et al. Acute stroke: improved nonenhanced CT detection—benefits of soft-copy interpretation by using variable window width and center level settings. *Radiology* 1999; **213**: 150–5.

3. Menon BK, Puetz V, Kochar P, Demchuk AM. ASPECTS and other neuroimaging scores in the triage and prediction of outcome in acute stroke patients. *Neuroimaging Clin N Am* 2011; **21**: 407–23, xii.

4. Pulli B, Schaefer PW, Hakimelahi R, et al. Acute ischemic stroke: infarct core estimation on CT angiography source images depends on CT angiography protocol. *Radiology* 2012; **262**: 593–604.

5. Souza LC, Yoo AJ, Chaudhry ZA, et al. Malignant CTA collateral profile is highly specific for large admission DWI infarct core and poor outcome in acute stroke. *AJNR Am J Neuroradiol* 2012; **33**: 1331–6.

6. Kamalian S, Maas MB, Goldmacher GV, et al. CT cerebral blood flow maps optimally correlate with admission diffusion-weighted imaging in acute stroke but thresholds vary by post-processing platform. *Stroke* 2011; **42**: 1923–8.

7. Dani KA, Thomas RG, Chappell FM, et al. Computed tomography and magnetic resonance perfusion imaging in ischemic stroke: definitions and thresholds. *Ann Neurol* 2011; **70**: 384–401.

8. Kidwell CS, Chalela JA, Saver JL, et al. Comparison of MRI and CT for detection of acute intracerebral hemorrhage. *JAMA* 2004; **292**: 1823–30.

9. Fiehler J, Albers GW, Boulanger JM, et al. Bleeding risk analysis in stroke imaging before thromboLysis (BRASIL): pooled analysis of T2*-weighted magnetic resonance imaging data from 570 patients. *Stroke* 2007; **38**: 2738–44.

10. Adams HP, Jr., del Zoppo G, Alberts MJ, et al. Guidelines for the early management of adults with ischemic stroke: a guideline from the American Heart Association/American Stroke Association Stroke Council, Clinical Cardiology Council, Cardiovascular Radiology and Intervention Council, and the Atherosclerotic Peripheral Vascular Disease and Quality of Care Outcomes in Research Interdisciplinary Working Groups: the American Academy of Neurology affirms the value of this guideline as an educational tool for neurologists. *Stroke* 2007; **38**: 1655–711.

11. Hacke W, Kaste M, Bluhmki E, et al. Thrombolysis with alteplase 3 to 4.5 hours after acute ischemic stroke. *N Engl J Med* 2008; **359**: 1317–29.

12. Riedel CH, Zimmermann P, Jensen-Kondering U, et al. The importance of size: successful recanalization by intravenous thrombolysis in acute anterior stroke depends on thrombus length. *Stroke* 2011; **42**: 1775–7.

13. Yoo AJ, Verduzco LA, Schaefer PW, et al. MRI-based selection for intra-arterial stroke therapy: value of pretreatment diffusion-weighted imaging lesion volume in selecting patients with acute stroke who will benefit from early recanalization. *Stroke* 2009; **40**: 2046–54.

14. Yoo AJ, Chaudhry ZA, Leslie-Mazwi TM, et al. Endovascular treatment of acute ischemic stroke: current indications. *Tech Vasc Interv Radiol* 2012; **15**: 33–40.

15. Hill MD, Rowley HA, Adler F, et al. Selection of acute ischemic stroke patients for intra-arterial thrombolysis with pro-urokinase by using ASPECTS. *Stroke* 2003; **34**: 1925–31.

16. Li Q, Lv F, Li Y, et al. Evaluation of 64-section CT angiography for detection and treatment planning of intracranial aneurysms by using DSA and surgical findings. *Radiology* 2009; **252**: 808–15.

17. Agid R, Andersson T, Almqvist H, et al. Negative CT angiography findings in patients with spontaneous subarachnoid hemorrhage: When is digital subtraction angiography still needed? *AJNR Am J Neuroradiol* 2010; **31**: 696–705.

18. Romero JM, Artunduaga M, Forero NP, et al. Accuracy of CT angiography for the diagnosis of vascular abnormalities causing intraparenchymal hemorrhage in young patients. *Emerg Radiol* 2009; **16**: 195–201.

19. Delgado Almandoz JE, Schaefer PW, Forero NP, et al. Diagnostic accuracy and yield of multidetector CT angiography in the evaluation of spontaneous intraparenchymal cerebral hemorrhage. *AJNR Am J Neuroradiol* 2009; **30**: 1213–21.

20. Zhu XL, Chan MS, Poon WS. Spontaneous intracranial hemorrhage: which patients need diagnostic cerebral angiography? A prospective study of 206 cases and review of the literature. *Stroke* 1997; **28**: 1406–9.

21. Delgado Almandoz JE, Yoo AJ, Stone MJ, et al. Systematic characterization of the computed tomography angiography spot sign in primary intracerebral hemorrhage identifies patients at highest risk for hematoma expansion: the spot sign score. *Stroke* 2009; **40**: 2994–3000.

3

Treatment of Acute Ischemic Stroke

Nader Antonios, MBChB, MPH&TM and Scott Silliman, MD

Department of Neurology, College of Medicine-Jacksonville, University of Florida, Jacksonville, FL

Introduction

When assessing a patient with an acute ischemic stroke, the question of whether or not they are a candidate for intravenous thrombolysis or an interventional procedure is often foremost in the clinician's mind. Factors such as time of symptom onset, stroke severity, associated medical conditions, and laboratory and radiographic findings play key roles in decision making. Patients must be carefully selected, based on available history and data, for acute stroke interventions in order to maximize potential benefit and minimize potential harm. Acquisition of information and its integration into a treatment plan must occur rapidly in order to meet targeted therapeutic windows. In this chapter, evidence supporting the use of intravenous thrombolysis, intra-arterial thrombolysis, and intra-arterial clot retrieval is reviewed. Patient selection criteria and challenging clinical circumstances where decision making may be difficult are also discussed.

Intravenous thrombolysis

Key clinical trials

Current treatment practices are based on two phase 3, multicenter, placebo-controlled trials. The National Institute of Neurological Disorders and Stroke (NINDS) sponsored study examined the safety and utility of recombinant tissue plasminogen activator (rt-PA) within a 3-hour window following acute ischemic stroke symptom onset. The results of this study, which were published in 1995, led to United States Food and Drug Administration (FDA) approval of the use of intravenous (IV) rt-PA for acute ischemic stroke [1]. The results of the European Cooperative Acute Stroke Study (ECASS) III study, published in 2008, support extension of the treatment window to 4.5 hours following symptom onset [2].

> ### ⚙ SCIENCE REVISITED
>
> Thrombi are comprised of an agglutination of red blood cells, platelets, and fibrin. Polymerized fibrin forms a mesh throughout and over a thrombus, which helps to solidify the thrombus. During thrombolysis, the fibrin component of a thrombus is fragmented by the enzyme plasmin. Breakdown of the fibrin mesh leads to thrombus dissolution. Within the normal physiologic thrombolytic cascade, plasmin is derived from plasminogen. Tissue plasminogen activator, which is secreted by damaged endothelial cells of blood vessels, catalyzes the conversion of plasminogen to plasmin. Tissue plasminogen activator is currently produced, for pharmacological use, via recombinant biotechnological methods. When administered intravenously or intra-arterially rt-PA can lyse emboli or thrombi that obstruct intracranial arteries and are responsible for inciting an ischemic stroke (Figure 3.1).

Stroke, First Edition. Edited by Kevin M. Barrett and James F. Meschia.
© 2013 John Wiley & Sons, Ltd. Published 2013 by John Wiley & Sons, Ltd.

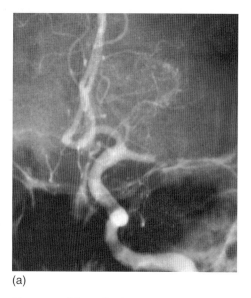
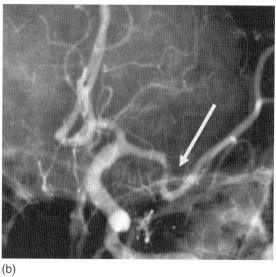

(a)   (b)

Figure 3.1 (a) Cerebral angiogram demonstrating occlusion of the left middle cerebral artery stem. (b) Repeat angiogram conducted several hours following administration of intravenous rt-PA demonstrates restoration of blood flow through the middle cerebral artery. There is residual partial obstruction of the middle cerebral artery stem (arrow).

NINDS rt-PA and ECASS III trials

The NINDS rt-PA study consisted of two parts. In Part 1, 291 patients with acute ischemic stroke were randomly assigned within 3 hours after symptom onset to either IV rt-PA (0.9 mg/kg with a maximal dose of 90 mg) or placebo. Strict inclusion and exclusion criteria were utilized to identify study subjects. The primary endpoint was the rate of complete neurologic recovery or neurologic improvement of at least 4 points on the National Institute of Health Stroke Scale (NIHSS) score at 24 hours. There was no significant difference in the percent of patients in the rt-PA-treated group (51%) and the placebo-treated group (46%) who attained this primary outcome (relative risk with rt-PA was 1.1; 95% confidence interval 0.8–1.6; $P = 0.56$).

In Part 2, 333 additional patients were randomized to either IV rt-PA (0.9 mg/kg with a maximal dose of 90 mg) or placebo; however, the primary endpoint was the rate of complete recovery or near complete recovery at 90 days. Four validated outcome scales were utilized in this study, with one scale measuring physical deficit (NIHSS), one scale measuring ability to conduct activities of daily living (Barthel Index (BI)) and two outcome measures assessing function (Modified Rankin Scale (mRS), Glasgow Outcome Scale). The rt-PA-treated patients were more likely to have favorable outcome assessed by all four measures (Table 3.1). In Part 2, a global test statistic that simultaneously tests for effect in all four outcome measures was utilized to conduct the primary outcome comparison between rt-PA and placebo-treated patients. The clinical benefit of rt-PA was confirmed by this analysis with a global odds ratio of 1.7 (95% CI, 1.2–2.6; $P = 0.008$).

The primary safety concern associated with rt-PA for treatment of acute ischemic stroke is symptomatic hemorrhagic transformation of cerebral infarction (SICH) (Figure 3.2). SICH occurred within 36 hours of treatment in 6.4% of IV rt-PA-treated patients and in 0.6% of placebo-treated patients (Table 3.1). One-half of the SICHs in the active treatment arm were fatal. Despite the tenfold higher risk of SICH, however, there was no significant difference in mortality between the two treatment groups at 3 months.

The ECASS III study examined the potential benefit of IV rt-PA administration for acute ischemic stroke between 3 and 4.5 hours after symptom onset. The study included 821 patients who were randomized to IV rt-PA (0.9 mg/kg with a maximal dose of 90 mg) or placebo. Clinical inclusion/

Table 3.1 Pivotal intravenous rt-PA trials

	NINDS Trial	ECASS III
Treatment window (hours)	0–3.0	3.0–4.5
rt-PA dose	0.9 mg/kg*	0.9 mg/kg*
Median baseline NIHSS	14 vs. 15 (NS)	10.7 vs. 11.6 (NS)
Patients with favorable outcome at 3 months: rt-PA vs. placebo (%)		
NIHSS 0 or 1	31 vs. 20	50 vs. 43
BI ≥95	50 vs. 38	63 vs. 59 (NS)
mRS 0 or 1	39 vs. 26	52 vs. 45
Glasgow Outcome Scale	44 vs. 32	
SICH: rt-PA vs. placebo (%)	6.4 vs. 0.6	2.4 vs. 0.2
Mortality at 3 months: rt-PA vs. placebo (%)	17 vs. 21 (NS)	8 vs. 8 (NS)

BI, Barthel Index; mRS, modified Rankin Scale; NIHSS, National Institute of Health Stroke Score; rt-PA, recombinant tissue plasminogen activator; SICH, symptomatic intracerebral hemorrhage; *Maximum dose = 90 mg.
All outcomes were statistically significantly different unless specified as NS.

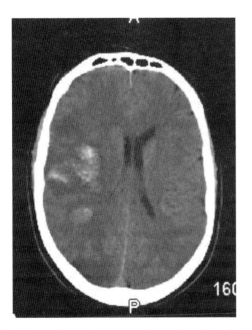

Figure 3.2 Hemorrhagic transformation of a right middle cerebral artery distribution ischemic stroke. The noncontrast head CT scan was performed 12 hours following the administration of intravenous rt-PA.

exclusion criteria were similar to the NINDS study except for the addition of the following exclusion criteria: (1) age >80 years; (2) NIHSS score >25; (3) oral anticoagulant use regardless of the international normalized ratio (INR); and (4) a history of combined prior stroke and diabetes (Table 3.2; Figure 3.3). Three outcome scales were utilized to assess patient outcome (mRS, NIHSS, BI). The primary outcome was disability at 90 days based on the mRS (Table 3.3) with favorable outcome pre-specified as an mRS 0–1, and score for unfavorable outcome was 2–6. Significantly more patients receiving IV rt-PA had a favorable outcome than patients treated with placebo (Table 3.1).

The incidence of symptomatic intracranial hemorrhage (2.4%) was tenfold higher than the incidence of symptomatic intracerebral hemorrhage in the placebo group (0.2%); however, the absolute risk was lower than the risk observed in the NINDS trial. Despite this risk of hemorrhage, there was no difference in mortality between the rt-PA-treated patients and the placebo group: 7.7% and 8.4%, respectively ($P = 0.68$).

Interpreting the NINDS and ECASS III studies

Outcomes in placebo-controlled intervention trials can be described in several ways. One way is to directly compare the percent of study subjects in the active treatment and placebo arms to discern the relative effectiveness of the study drug. When utilizing this comparison, rt-PA-treated patients in the NINDS study were 55% more likely than placebo-treated patients to have the primary outcome of an NIHSS of 0–1 at 3 months (31% with this outcome in the treated arm vs. 20% in the placebo arm). In the ECASS III trial, rt-PA-treated patients were 16% more likely than placebo-treated patients

Table 3.2 Inclusion and exclusion criteria for the intravenous administration of intravenous rt-PA between 3 and 4.5 hours following stroke onset

Inclusion

Infusion can begin within 3 hours of symptom onset

NIHSS ≥4*

Baseline CT scan shows no intracranial hemorrhage, mass lesion responsible for symptoms, or an early hypodensity affecting ≥ one-third of a middle cerebral artery territory†

Exclusion

History of another stroke or serious head trauma within the preceding 3 months

Age >80 years of age

NIHSS score >25

Current oral anticoagulant use regardless of the normalized ratio (INR)

A history of combined prior stroke and diabetes

Major surgery within 14 days

History of intracranial hemorrhage*

Systolic blood pressure (BP) >185 mmHg or diastolic BP >110 mmHg and aggressive treatment required to reduce blood pressure to these limits BP*

Rapidly improving or minor symptoms*

Seizure at the onset of stroke*

Symptoms suggestive of subarachnoid hemorrhage (SAH) despite negative CT

Gastrointestinal hemorrhage or urinary tract hemorrhage within the previous 21 days

Arterial puncture at a noncompressible site within the previous 7 days

Administration of heparin within 48 hours preceding the onset of stroke, with an activated partial thromboplastin time exceeding the upper limit of the normal range

Platelet counts <100,000/μL

Glucose level <50/dl mg and symptoms improve following dextrose administration or glucose >400/dl mg per deciliter and treating physician believes these symptoms are by induced hyperglycemia

*See "Optimizing Clinical Outcomes" section of this chapter for discussion on flexible interpretation based on clinical scenario.

†See Figure 3.3 for an example of this radiographic finding.

to have the primary outcome of a MRS of 0,1 at 3 months (52% with this outcome in the treated arm vs. 45% in the placebo arm).

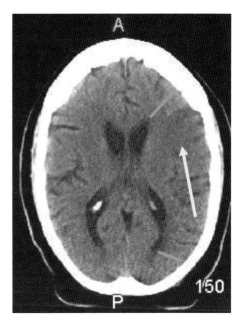

Figure 3.3 Noncontrast head CT conducted in a patient 3.5 hours following symptom onset. The CT demonstrated an early hypodensity of the left middle cerebral artery territory affecting more than one-third of the middle cerebral artery territory. The middle cerebral artery is demarcated by the lines. Note the hypodense region within the anterior half of this arterial territory. Due to this finding, the patient was not a candidate for intravenous rt-PA. There is also blurring of the gray matter/white matter boundary of the left frontal cortex (arrow).

A more accurate way of interpreting the effectiveness of a health-care intervention is to evaluate the number of patients who need to be treated with the intervention to achieve one beneficial outcome. This numerical value, termed "number needed to treat" (NNT), is the inverse of the absolute risk reduction produced by the intervention as compared with placebo. A lower NNT is indicative of a more effective treatment. In the NINDS trial the average absolute risk reduction among the four outcome measures is 12. Thus, within the 0 to 3-hour window, 8.5 patients need to be treated with rt-PA to achieve an additional good outcome. Within the 3 to 4.5-hour treatment examined in the ECASS III trial, rt-PA treatment was associated with a 7% higher likelihood of achieving the primary outcome of an mRS 0–1 compared with placebo. The number needed to treat with rt-PA in the 3 to 4.5-hour treatment window is 14.

Table 3.3 Modified Rankin score

Score	Definition
0	No symptoms
1	No significant disability. Able to carry out all usual activities, despite some symptoms.
2	Slight disability. Able to look after own affairs without assistance, but unable to carry out all previous activities.
3	Moderate disability. Requires some help, but able to walk unassisted.
4	Moderately severe disability. Unable to attend to own bodily needs without assistance, and unable to walk unassisted.
5	Severe disability. Requires constant nursing care and attention, bedridden, incontinent.
6	Death

A Modified Rankin Score of 0 or 1 at 3 months post rt-PA or placebo treatment was considered to be favorable outcome in the NINDS and the ECASS III studies. In the PROACT II study, an MRS of ≤2 was considered to be favorable outcome.

those patients who are eligible for treatment in the 3 to 4.5-hour time window, "Treatment with tPA is associated with a 9 in 20 chance of having no significant disability at 3 months. Without treatment the chance of having no significant disability at 3 month is 11 in 20."

Safety of a therapeutic intervention can be described by the "number needed to harm" (NNH). This measure indicates how many patients need to be exposed to an intervention to cause harm in one additional patient. This number is the inverse of the attributable risk. In the NINDS study, rt-PA treatment produced an attributable risk of symptomatic intracerebral hemorrhage of 5.8% (6.4% in rt-PA-treated patients vs. 0.6% in placebo-treated patients). The corresponding NNH is 17. In the ECASS III study, rt-PA treatment was associated with an attributable risk of symptomatic hemorrhagic infarction of 2.2% (2.4% in rt-PA-treated patients vs. 0.2% in placebo-treated patients). The corresponding NNH is 45.

☆ TRICKS AND TIPS

Discussion of the potential benefits of rt-PA is a key element of the informed consent process prior to rt-PA administration. An accurate understanding of the potential benefits by the patient and/or their family may be difficult. Factors such as stroke-induced language dysfunction, health literacy level, and inattention occurring during a stressful event can contribute to poor comprehension and retention of information concerning rt-PA efficacy. Discussing the potential benefit of treatment in absolute terms rather than in relative terms may provide clarity prior to consent for treatment. For example, "Treatment with tPA is associated with a 1 in 3 chance of having a normal or near normal neurologic exam at 3 months. Without treatment the chance of having a normal or near normal neurologic exam is 1 in 5." is an accurate and comprehendible way to convey rt-PA efficacy to candidates for treatment within 3 hours of symptom onset. Similarly, for

☆ TIPS AND TRICKS

The risk of symptomatic hemorrhagic transformation associated with rt-PA treatment must be included as part of the informed consent process. Discussing the risk by utilizing a direct comparison, rather than a relative comparison, is easiest for patients to understand. Consent to treat discussions must also incorporate information regarding the risk of death following hemorrhagic transformation. For those patients in whom treatment is being contemplated within 3 hours, an example of a way to convey this information is: "The risk of tPA causing bleeding in the brain is 1 in 16 whereas routine treatment without tPA is associated with a 1 in 166 risk of bleeding. Half of the bleeds produced by tPA are ultimately fatal, however if a bleed occurs there are medical and surgical treatment options that we consider to potentially reduce the risk of a bad outcome." Obviously, the risk of hemorrhagic transformation can be daunting information for a patient or their family to hear. The clinician must convey that the risk is incorporated into the favorable outcome data, and that the overall risk of death following rt-PA administration at 3 months following stroke onset is no different in patients treated with rt-PA than in patients not treated with rt-PA (Table 3.1). For those patients being considered for treatment in the 3 to 4.5-hour window, the physician can convey that "the risk of tPA causing bleeding in the brain is 1 in 40 whereas no treatment is associated with a 1 in 500 risk. This hemorrhage can cause worsening of symptoms or be fatal. The risk of death by 3 months from this time point, however, is no different if we proceed with tPA treatment versus not treating with tPA."

Differences in efficacy and safety outcomes in the NINDS and ECASS III trials

The lower NNT observed in the NINDS trial is likely explained by biologic factors associated with the earlier treatment window in the NINDS trial. Patients in this trial were treated, on average, almost 2 hours earlier than in the ECASS III trial. Therefore, a higher percentage of neurons in the ischemic zone become irreversibly damaged and are destroyed when treatment is initiated later. The lower NNH demonstrated in the NINDS trial probably relates to differences in patient selection criteria utilized in the two trials. Two exclusion criterion used in ECASS III, namely history of diabetes mellitus plus prior ischemic stroke and warfarin use regardless of INR, were incorporated into the protocol specifically to help minimize risk of hemorrhagic transformation. In addition, average infarction size was smaller in ECASS III than in the NINDS trial. This difference in infarct size is exemplified by the lower median baseline NIHSS in the ECASS III trial than in the NINDS Trial (Table 3.1). Small infarctions are less likely to undergo hemorrhagic transformation than large infarctions. The lower median NIHSS score in ECASS III was due to an exclusion cutoff of NIHSS >25 and exclusion of warfarin-treated patients. Warfarin is often utilized for ischemic stroke prophylaxis in patients with atrial fibrillation. Cardioembolic ischemic strokes associated with

atrial fibrillation tend to be larger than ischemic strokes induced by other mechanisms. Fewer patients with atrial fibrillation were enrolled into the rt-PA treatment arm of the ECASS III trial than the NINDS trial (12.7% vs. 20%).

Optimizing clinical outcomes following intravenous thrombolysis

Patient selection for treatment with IV rt-PA plays a key role in helping to ensure that individual outcomes following treatment parallel the outcomes achieved in the pivotal clinical trials. In addition, adherence to treatment inclusion/exclusion criteria and post-thrombolysis ancillary care reduce the risk of SICH. Exclusion criteria were absolute when utilized to screen patients for inclusion in the NINDS and ECASS III trials. In clinical practice, however, the only truly *absolute* contraindication to treatment with rt-PA is the presence of a hemorrhage on the baseline CT scan. Since publication of these trials, some of the exclusion criteria utilized in the trials have been refined based on expert consensus (Tables 3.2 and 3.4; Figure 3.3). These modified criteria should be interpreted, with a degree of flexibility, in the context of the specific clinical presentation of the individual:

- *NIHSS <4*: some deficits produced by brain infarction can be quite disabling despite being associated with a low NIHSS. For example an isolated homonymous hemianopsia produced by posterior cerebral artery distribution ischemia (NIHSS = 2) or an isolated severe expressive aphasia (NIHSS = 3) produced by middle cerebral artery branch ischemia can be disabling to many patients, particularly if the deficit threatens their ability to be employed and/or function independently.
- *Rapidly improving deficits*: patients with rapid and near-complete resolution of deficits may be exposed to the potential risks of rt-PA that outweigh the potential benefits of thrombolysis. Patients with waxing and waning symptoms or those with only slight improvement over the first hour should still be considered for rt-PA treatment. In addition, patients with an initial high NIHSS who improve, but still have an NIHSS >4 prior to the 3-hour time mark, should be considered for treatment as these patients are unlikely to have transient brain ischemia.

This point is exemplified by the fact that only 2% of placebo-treated patients in the NINDS trial with a deficit present at 3 hours following symptom onset had no neurological deficit at 24 hours.

- *History of intracerebral hemorrhage*: prior history of an intracerebral hemorrhage that was due to a condition associated with recurrent hemorrhages (e.g. rupture of a vascular malformation, primary intracerebral hemorrhage related to chronic hypertension, or amyloid angiopathy) excludes a patient from receiving rt-PA. Intracerebral hemorrhage that was not due to a recurrent condition (e.g. a remote history of traumatic subdural or epidural hematoma) should not exclude a patient provided that the baseline brain CT scan shows no residual hemorrhage.

- *Seizure at onset of stroke*: seizure at onset of stroke excluded enrollment into the NINDS rt-PA and ECASS III trials. This exclusion was included in the trial protocols to avoid enrollment of patients with neurological deficits caused postictal brain dysfunction. Seizures infrequently accompany acute brain ischemia. Clinicians can consider administrating intravenous rt-PA to patients with clinical or radiographic evidence suggestive of ischemic stroke. For example, a patient with a known severe left internal carotid artery stenosis and no history of prior seizures presenting with a postseizure aphasia and right hemiparesis may be an appropriate candidate for rt-PA. Use of emergent vascular imaging, such as CT or MR angiography, to demonstrate an intracranial arterial occlusion can be helpful in this scenario.

It has been estimated that the typical stroke patient loses nearly 2 million neurons each minute the stroke is untreated. Patients treated earlier within the window for intravenous thrombolysis have a better chance for favorable outcome than patients with a similar NIHSS who are treated later in the therapeutic window. Guidelines recommend a door-to-needle time of ≤60 minutes [3]. Currently, however, less than one-third of acute ischemic stroke patients who are treated with rt-PA are treated within this time frame. A combination of prehospital notification, single call stroke team activation, rapid completion and interpretation of brain

Table 3.4 Inclusion and exclusion criteria for the intravenous administration of rt-PA between 0 and 3 hours following stroke onset

Inclusion
Infusion can begin within 3 hours of symptom onset
NIHSS ≥4*
Baseline CT scan shows no intracranial hemorrhage, mass lesion responsible for symptoms, or an early hypodensity affecting ≥ one-third of a middle cerebral artery territory†

Exclusion
History of another stroke or serious head trauma within the preceding 3 months
Major surgery within 14 days
History of intracranial hemorrhage*
Systolic blood pressure (BP) >185 mmHg or diastolic BP >110 mmHg and aggressive treatment required to reduce blood pressure to these limits BP*
Rapidly improving or minor symptoms*
Seizure at the onset of stroke*
Symptoms suggestive of subarachnoid hemorrhage (SAH) despite negative CT
Gastrointestinal hemorrhage or urinary tract hemorrhage within the previous 21 days
Arterial puncture at a noncompressible site within the previous 7 days
Protime INR ≤1.7 seconds
Heparin use within the 48 hours preceding the onset of stroke with elevated PTT
Platelet counts <100,000/μL
Glucose level <50 mg/dL and symptoms improve following dextrose administration or glucose >400 mg/dL per deciliter and treating physician believes these symptoms are induced hyperglycemia

These contemporary criteria include modification of some of the original criteria utilized in the NINDS study . Modifications have occurred, over time, based on expert consensus opinion [3].
*See "Optimizing Clinical Outcomes" section of this chapter for discussion on flexible interpretation based on clinical scenario.
†See Figure 3.3 for an example of this radiographic finding.

imaging, use of standardized orders, and ongoing stroke team education with performance improvement feedback is recommended to help maximize the number of patients treated within 60 minutes of emergency department arrival.

★ TIPS AND TRICKS

In some cases, waiting for the results of the prothrombin time and partial thromboplastin time (PT and PTT) and/or the platelet count may threaten to push the rt-PA treatment window beyond the recommend limit of 3 hours or 4.5 hours. In such situations rt-PA can be administered prior to receipt of the coagulation test results if the patient has no clinical or historical factors that increase the risk of coagualopathy or thrombocytopenia. These factors include current use of warfarin, heparin, or heparinoid compounds, hemodialyis for endstage renal disease, hepatic disease, alcoholism, or active cancer.

Use of a standardized checklist to evaluate inclusion and exclusion criteria can speed the process of evaluating patients for rt-PA treatment. Standardized order sets for rt-PA administration and postadministration orders can also help to minimize delays associated with drug administration and postadministration transfer to a critical care unit.

Post-thrombolysis care

Following rt-PA infusion patients should be monitored in a critical care or stroke unit setting for at least 24 hours. Critical care or stroke units provide the advantage of close neurological observation and frequent blood pressure measurements. Key points regarding care during the first 24 hours following rt-PA infusion are:

- Blood pressure monitoring every 15 minutes during the infusion and the subsequent 2 hours, every 30 minutes for 6 hours, and every 60 minutes for the following 16 hours.
- If systolic blood pressure exceeds 180 mmHg or diastolic blood pressure exceeds 105 mmHg during the post-thrombolysis monitoring period, treatment of blood pressure with short-acting intravenous antihypertensive drugs such as labetalol (10 mg IV over 1–2 minutes; may repeat every 10–20 minutes with maximal dose 300 mg) should be initiated. If blood pressure fails to respond to adequate doses of labetalol, a continuous antihypertensive drug drip should be initiated (labetalol 2–8 mg/minute or nicardipine 5 mg/hour and titrate to goal blood pressure by increasing 2.5 mg/hour every 5 minutes to a maximum dose of 15 mg/hour).
- Obtain noncontrast brain CT at hour 24 +/– 8 hours to evaluate for hemorrhagic transformation.
- Do not initiate a secondary stroke prevention drug (aspirin, clodipigrel, Aggrenox, intravenous or low-molecular-weight heparin, or warfarin until the results of the 24-hour CT scan are known and integrated into decision making.
- Avoid subcutaneous heparin or low-molecular-weight heparin for deep venous thrombosis prophylaxis until the results of the 24-hour CT scan are known.
- Use sequential compression devices for deep venous thrombosis prophylaxis when subcutaneous heparin and low-molecular-weight heparin cannot be used.

Treating complications of rt-PA

The two primary complications associated with rt-PA are anaphylaxis and hemorrhage. Risk of symptomatic intracranial hemorrhage was discussed earlier in this chapter. Rarely, significant extracranial bleeding, such as gastrointestinal tract and oropharyngeal hemorrhage, occurs during or soon after drug infusion has been completed. If significant extracranial hemorrhage or symptomatic intracranial hemorrhage occurs, the following steps should be taken:

- If rt-PA is still being infused, discontinue the infusion.
- Type and cross match blood if a systemic hemorrhage has occurred.
- Treat with cryoprecipitate (10 units).
- For symptomatic intracranial hemorrhagic transformation, neurosurgical evaluation regarding feasibility and utility of a surgical intervention should be requested.

Allergic reactions such as anaphylactic reactions, orolingual edema, and rash may rarely occur. Orolingual angioedema is usually mild in severity and brief in duration; however, it can sometimes produce life-threatening airway compromise requiring intubation. Concurrent use of angiotensin converting enzyme (ACE) inhibitors increases the risk of this reaction. Orolingual angioedema has been attributed to increased bradykinin production. Tissue plasminogen activator converts plasminogen to plasmin, and plasmin cleaves bradykinin from kininogen. In some instances the lingual edema may involve only half of the tongue, with the involved side being contralateral to the cerebral hemisphere affected by brain ischemia. Treatment of anaphylaxis and orolingual edema involves immediate airway evaluation and management should proceed appropriately according to the airway status. Intravenous administration of a single dose of methylprednisolone (250–1000 mg) or antihistamine (e.g. clemastine 2 mg) should be considered. Icatibant (bradykinin B2 receptor antagonist) administered as a subcutaneous single injection (30 mg) may be potentially an effective therapy. ACE inhibitors should be discontinued. If possible, treatment with epinephrine should be avoided due to its propensity to raise blood pressure; thus theoretically its use may increase risk of hemorrhagic transformation of the stroke.

Special patient circumstances

The presence of certain clinical circumstances with an acute ischemic stroke can make the decision to treat a patient with intravenous rt-PA complex. These cases may present a challenge to the clinician and the decision to administer rt-PA should be individualized. In these situations, a patient may wish to accept the risk of treatment over the risk of having a persistent disabling neurologic deficit. Discussion of some of these circumstances follows.

Pregnancy

The safety of intravenous rt-PA in pregnant women with acute ischemic stroke is unknown since pregnant women were excluded from clinical trials of thrombolytic drugs. Case reports of successful treatment of pregnant women have been published. Intravenous rt-PA does not cross the placenta and there is no documented evidence of teratogenicity in animal models. The primary concern of administering rt-PA during pregnancy is the potential risk of fetal hemorrhage, maternal hemorrhage, or placental abruption. rt-PA is a category C medication, that is its safety is uncertain in pregnancy. The package insert indicates that it "should be used during pregnancy only if the potential benefit justifies the potential risk to the fetus." For example, it may be justified to treat a pregnant woman who has experienced a dominant hemisphere global middle

cerebral artery syndrome provided that her legally authorized representative understands the potential risks and consents to treatment.

Cervical arterial dissection

There are no adequate randomized trials to definitely determine the safety and efficacy of intravenous rt-PA in the setting of arterial dissection. Arterial dissection was not included in the eligibility criteria of the large thrombolysis trials. Thrombolysis in cervical arterial dissection carries the theoretical risk of intramural hematoma extension and new or progressive compression of lower cranial nerves, progressive luminal narrowing, vessel rupture, dislocation of intraluminal thrombus with subsequent arterial embolism, subarachnoid hemorrhage related to intracranial extension of the dissection, or pseudoaneurysm formation. Case reports suggest that these risks are low. Thrombolysis should not be considered a contraindication in patients with suspected cervical arterial dissection.

Aortic dissection

Approximately 5% of thoracic aortic dissections are associated with cerebral embolism. The mechanism for cerebral embolism is likely related to aortogenic emboli or emboli originating in cervical arteries propagating distally. Clinicians should consider the presence of aortic dissection when chest and/or upper back pain occurs as part of an acute stroke syndrome. Chest pain may not be reported by patients with acute aphasia related to cerebral infarction, which makes the diagnosis of aortic dissection difficult in patients with large dominant hemisphere infarctions. The chest X-ray usually shows mediastinal widening; however, it may be negative in 20% of cases. The diagnosis can be confirmed by computed tomography of the chest. Although, aortic dissection was not included as an exclusion criterion in the NINDS or ECASS III trials, it is generally considered a contraindication for IV thrombolysis in acute ischemic stroke. Thrombolysis of patients with aortic dissection carries possible risks such as aortic rupture, hemothorax, and hemopericardium. In addition, administration of rt-PA is also likely to delay emergent cardiothoracic surgical procedures. There are no adequate studies that delineate the absolute frequency and magnitude of complications following intravenous thrombolysis in the presence of aortic dissection.

⚠ CAUTION

Intravenous thrombolysis should be avoided in acute ischemic stroke associated with aortic dissection due to the high potential to cause serious harm to the patient.

Infectious endocarditis

Endocarditis is a microbial infection of the intracardiac structures. The most common etiology of infectious endocarditis is bacterial. Fungal infections account for a small minority of cases. Stroke is the most frequent neurologic complication of infectious endocarditis, with stroke occurring in nearly one-third of cases. Ischemic stroke in the setting of infectious endocarditis is presumed to be due to septic cardiogenic embolism. Embolic stroke is one of the most frequent presenting medical events associated with infectious endocarditis. Hemorrhagic transformation of acute septic embolic infarctions is not infrequent and relates to septic arteritis with vascular wall erosion.

There are limited safety data regarding the use of thrombolysis in patient with acute ischemic stroke related to bacterial endocarditis. Case reports of intracranial hemorrhages occurring in patients with infective endocarditis treated with thrombolytic agents for acute coronary syndrome have been published.

⚠ CAUTION

In view of the potential for hemorrhagic complications in patients with ischemic stroke due to septic embolism, it is prudent not to administer rt-PA to patients with known or suspected infective endocarditis.

Pediatric stroke

Patients <18 years old were excluded from the NINDS and ECASS III studies and results from randomized clinical trials of the efficacy and safety of thrombolysis in this age group do not exist. Adult guidelines for administration of rt-PA cannot be extrapolated to children due to differences in brain development and recovery from brain insults, coagulation systems, and stroke etiologies between children and adults. Treatment may be justified in some older adolescents with severe strokes who meet standard adult criteria for rt-PA therapy.

Endovascular arterial reperfusion

Acute occlusion of a large intracranial artery such as the carotid terminus, middle cerebral, vertebral, basilar, anterior cerebral, and posterior cerebral arteries are often associated with poor outcomes. Proximal vascular occlusions represent the primary targets for direct intra-arterial endovascular reperfusion therapies. Currently, two endovascular reperfusion strategies exist: intra-arterial thrombolysis (IAT) and mechanical thrombectomy. IAT involves direct administration of a fibrinolytic drug into a thrombus or embolus via a catheter delivery system (Figure 3.4). Mechanical thrombectomy entails extraction of a thrombus or an embolus with a catheter-based device. These intra-arterial therapies are applicable to a subset of patients with acute brain ischemia induced by intracranial large artery occlusion, particularly in situations when patients are beyond a time limit for IV rt-PA or have a specific exclusion to IV rt-PA. In this section of the chapter key clinical trials, inclusion/ exclusion criteria, and efficacy associated with the different IAT procedures are reviewed.

Key clinical trials of intra-arterial thrombolysis

PROACT II, published in 1998, is the only completed phase 3 clinical trial of intra-arterial thrombolysis [4]. This study was a multicenter, randomized, open-label clinical trial with blinded follow-up involving 180 patients at 54 centers in the USA and Canada. Patients were randomized to receive local intra-arterial (IA) recombinant prourokinase (9 mg over 120 min) plus low-dose IV heparin (2000 IU bolus with 500 IU/hour for 4 hours) (n=121) versus low-dose IV heparin alone (n=59). Key inclusion and exclusion criteria are given in Table 3.5. Patients with an NIHSS <4 were not considered candidates for study entry because they usually have a favorable prognosis and the low likelihood of having a middle cerebral artery occlusion. All subjects had repeat angiography to assess recanalization. The primary outcome measure was the proportion of patients with minimal or no neurologic disability at 90 days, as defined by a modified Rankin score of 2 or less. Significantly more patients in the prourokinase arm achieved the primary outcome measure (Table 3.6).

Despite the increased frequency of symptomatic hemorrhagic transformation, overall mortality was not different in the two arms (prourokinase 25% vs.

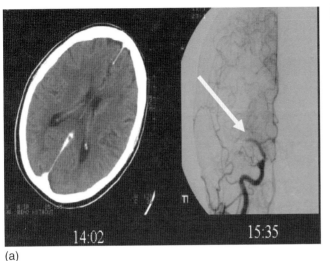
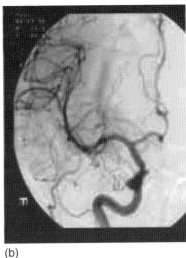

(a)   (b)

Figure 3.4 (a) Baseline noncontrast head CT scan and cerebral angiogram in a patient with a proximal right middle cerebral artery stem occlusion (arrow). CT scan is normal. Angiographic picture was obtained 93 minutes following completion of noncontrast CT. (b) Recanalizations of the right middle cerebral artery stem occlusion following treatment with intra-arterial rt-PA. This angiographic picture was obtained 178 minutes following completion of the CT scan.

Table 3.5 PROACT II inclusion/exclusion criteria: intra-arterial thrombolysis for acute ischemic stroke

Inclusion
> Acute ischemic stroke symptoms <6 hours duration and start of infusion can occur prior within 6 hours
> NIHSS ≥4
> Disabling or life threatening stroke
> Angiographic evidence of middle cerebral artery (MCA) stem or division occlusion

Exclusion
> Evidence of hemorrhage or mass on noncontrast head CT or brain MRI
> History of intracerebral hemorrhage or subarachnoid hemorrhage*
> Bleeding diathesis
> International normalized ratio ≥1.7
> Thrombocytopenia: platelets ≤ 100,000 cells/µL

These criteria were utilized in the PROACT II trial that evaluated the efficacy and safety of pro-urokinase for intra-arterial thrombolysis. These inclusion and exclusion criteria have been widely extrapolated and applied as selection criteria for patients who are candidates for intra-arterial thrombolysis with rt-PA [3]. Enrollment into the PROACT II trial was limited to patients with MCA stem or division occlusion. In current clinical practice intra-arterial thrombolysis is also considered, in appropriate patients, with a symptomatic occlusion of another major intracranial artery.

*History of intracerebral hemorrhage was an absolute exclusion for patient enrollment into the PROACT II Study. In clinical practice, however, history of intracerebral hemorrhage is not an absolute contraindication to conducting intra-arterial thrombolysis. Patients with a prior intracerebral hemorrhage that was not due to a recurrent condition (i.e. a remote history of traumatic subdural or epidural hematoma) should not be excluded provided that the baseline brain CT scan shows no residual hemorrhage.

control 27%). Although the results of this study were positive, the study did not result in FDA approval of prourokinase or IAT. As of 2012, there are no FDA approved drugs for use in IAT and prourokinase is not commercially available in the United States. Recombinant t-PA is currently used as the fibrinolytic drug for IAT, however intra-arterial administration of rt-PA for treatment of acute ischemic

Table 3.6 Prospective endovascular arterial reperfusion trials

	Proact II	MERCI*	Multi-Merci*	Penumbra*
Treatment type	IA pUK + Hep vs. Hep	IA Merci + IAT	IA Merci + IAT + IVT	IA Pen + IAT
Patients	180 (121 vs. 59)	141	164	125
Time window (hours)	0–6	0–8	0–8	0–8
Mean baseline NIHSS	17 vs. 17	20	19	17
Recanalization (%)	66 vs. 18	60.3	68	81.6
		(48 device alone)	(55 device alone)	(device alone)
Outcome (%) at 3 months mRS <2	40 vs. 25	36	36	25
SICH rate (%)	10 vs. 2	7.8	9.8	11.2

*Historical controls were used as the comparison arm for these clinical trials – a concurrent control group was not included in the study design.

IA, intra-arterial; IAT, intra-arterial therapy; IVT, intravenous thrombolysis; NIHSS, National Institutes of Health Stroke Scale; mRS, Modified Rankin Scale; SICH, symptomatic intracerebral hemorrhage.

stroke has not been subjected to clinical trials. Intra-arterial therapy should be considered only when there are adequate personnel and facilities to ensure appropriate patient selection, and procedural and postprocedural care. The American Heart Association/ American Stroke Association guidelines for stroke management recommend off-label IAT with rt-PA for selected patients who present within 6 hours following stroke onset and are not candidates for IV rt-PA. This recommendation comes with the caveat that there is insufficient trial evidence to recommend the optimal IAT agent, dose, or delivery technique and that the availability of intra-arterial thrombolysis should not preclude the intravenous administration of rt-PA in otherwise eligible patients [4].

> ### ⚗ SCIENCE REVISITED
>
> Urokinase is a naturally occurring protease that is manufactured by uroendothelial cells. Urokinase, like rt-PA, converts plasminogen to plasmin. Prourokinase is a proenzyme that remains inactive in the absence of fibrin and is not activated in circulating blood. It is activated by plasmin at the site of thrombosis. Since it is not active in circulating blood, the thrombolytic activity of prourokinase is restricted to the embolus or thrombus obstructing an artery. Prourokinase utilized in the PROACT II Study was manufactured with recombinant technology.

Special clinical scenario: acute basilar artery occlusion

Clinical outcomes documented in series of patients with angiographically demonstrated basilar artery occlusions suggest a high case fatality rate and poor neurological outcome in survivors. Benign outcome, without interventional thrombolysis, is most often associated with short segment basilar occlusions of mostly atherothrombotic origin in patients with good collateral supply. An IAT approach to treating acute basilar artery occlusion has not been the subject of a randomized clinical trial comparing it to a medical therapy or intravenous thrombolysis. It is unlikely that any large-scale randomized clinical trials of intra-arterial therapy will be conducted in patients with basilar occlusion.

Single-center case series suggest that interventional thrombolysis can reduce mortality and improve outcome in selected patients (Table 3.7). In these single-center experiences, treatment windows have been longer than those utilized for intra-arterial recanalization in the anterior circulation. This longer window relates to the lower likelihood of SICH in the posterior circulation and the possibility that brainstem structures may be more resistant to ischemia than the cerebral white matter and cortical tissue. Exceptional cases of good recovery with treatment as late as 12 hours or more have been reported. Even with successful recanalization of the basilar artery, however, there is still an approximately 50% mortality rate.

Table 3.7 Representative case series of intra-arterial thrombolysis for basilar artery occlusion

	Brandt et al. [5]	Jung et al. [6]
Patients	51	106
Fibrinolytic drug	urokinase: 44	urokinase: 58
	tPA: 9	urokinase + mechanical: 33
		mechanical only: 15
Mean time to treatment (minutes)	502	330
Recanalization (%)	51	70
Mortality	46% with recanalization 92% without recanalization	41%
Good neurological outcome	10/16 survivors BI ≥95	33% with mRS 0–2
SICH rate (%)	0	1

tPA, tissue plasminogen activator; BI: Barthel Index; mRS: Modified Rankin Scale; SICH: symptomatic intracerebral hemorrhage.

Following the advent of mechanical thrombectomy, IAT is sometimes combined with these mechanical techniques to augment reperfusion of the basilar artery.

Decisions to treat must be determined on a case-by-case basis utilizing available clinical and radiologic data and on the availability of the necessary interventional resources. A therapeutic response in patients with coma and clinical examination of diffuse brainstem damage, including bilateral fixed and dilated pupils is, unlikely. Clearly defined areas of brainstem or cerebellar infarction detected on CT imaging or T2 MRI sequences are unlikely to respond to thrombolysis. Because no randomized trials have been performed to establish the safety of and efficacy of reperfusion in posterior circulation strokes, the procedure should be reserved for patients with progressive, disabling, or life-threatening brainstem strokes if the clinician believes there is a reasonable potential for clinically meaningful recovery.

Mechanical thrombectomy

Mechanical thrombectomy devices that have received US Food and Drug Administration clearance and are currently utilized in clinical practice are the Merci Retriever (Concentric Medical, Mountain View, California) the Penumbra System (Penumbra, Alameda, California), and the Solitaire device (Covidien, Mansfield, Massachusetts) which are indicated for use within 8 hours of symptom onset in patients with large intracranial vessel occlusion.

Merci Retriever

The Concentric MERCI (Mechanical Embolus Removal in Cerebral Ischemia) Retrieval System is a corkscrew-like apparatus designed to remove clots from vessels in patients experiencing an ischemic stroke. The corkscrew resides in the catheter tip, which shields it from the arterial wall until it is ready to be deployed into the clot. Once buried in the clot, the device and clot are withdrawn from the artery. The first generation models (X5 and X6) were approved for commercial use in 2004. The MERCI Retriever has received approval from the US Food and Drug Administration (FDA) for use in patients with persistent vessel occlusion after IV rt-PA. The FDA has approved the MERCI device for reopening intracranial arteries in acute ischemic stroke. Its clinical efficacy, however, has not been fully established in a controlled outcomes trial evaluating it against another intra-arterial reperfusion therapy. Since this device has not been compared directly to intravenous or an untreated control group, its precise utility in improving outcomes after stroke remains unclear. A video demonstrating its deployment can be viewed at: http://www.youtube.com/watch?v=P2TNz-TniIA.

Key clinical trials

Two clinical trials evaluating the efficacy of this device have been published. Both studies were prospective, multicenter, single-armed studies with historical controls. In the Mechanical Embolus Removal in Cerebral Embolism (MERCI) trial, vessels

Table 3.8 Clinical characteristics of patients who are candidates for Merci or Multi-Merci

Inclusion

Stroke symptom duration <8 hours

Contraindication for IV tPA if stroke symptom duration <4.5 hours or IV rt-PA cannot be infused by hour 4.5 if no contraindications exist

NIHSS score ≥8

Cerebral angiography demonstrating occlusion of a treatable vessel (intracranial vertebral artery, basilar artery, intracranial carotid artery (ICA), ICA terminal bifurcation, the middle cerebral artery (MCA) first division (M1), or an occlusion of the division of the MCA (M2)

Exclusion

Excessive tortuosity of cervical vessels precluding device delivery

Known hemorrhagic diathesis or known coagulation factor deficiency

Oral anticoagulation treatment with international normalized ratio >3.0

Use of heparin within 48 hours, and a partial thromboplastin time (PTT) >2 times normal

Platelet count <50,000/μL

History of severe allergy to contrast media

Sustained systolic blood pressure >185 mmHg or diastolic blood pressure >110 mmHg despite treatment

CT scan revealing significant mass effect with midline shift or greater than one-third of the MCA region with hypodensity (sulcal effacement and/or loss of gray–white differentiation alone was allowed)

>50% stenosis of the artery proximal to the target vessel

Life expectancy <3 months

The criteria utilized in the Merci and Multi-Merci trails were similar with the exceptions that: (1) platelet count <30,000/μL was an exclusion in Multi Merci and <50,000/μL was an exclusion in the Merci Trial; (2) patients with an M2 MCA occlusion were not included in the Merci Trial but were eligible for enrollment into the Multi-Merci trial; and (3) INR >1.7 excluded enrollment into the Merci trial whereas INR >3.0 excluded enrollment into the Multi-Merci Trial. The Merci and Multi-Merci trials only enrolled patients with symptoms between 3 and 8 hours' duration.

were opened within 8 hours from symptom onset with a device that removed the thrombus from an intracranial artery [7]. Inclusion and exclusion criteria (Table 3.8) utilized in this trial are similar to those utilized in the PROACT II trial. Notable inclusion differences, however, are a longer treatment window (8 hours from stroke onset), higher allowable INR (3.0), and a higher NIHSS minimal score (8). Rapid opening of the artery was achieved, but overall efficacy and safety achieved with the MERCI retrieval system were similar to those that occurred with intra-arterial prourokinase in the PROACT-II trial. For instance, the rate of recanalization of the middle cerebral artery in MERCI was 45%, and it was 66% in PROACT-II (Table 3.6). In the MERCI trial, 17 patients received thrombolytic medications when the device was unable to achieve adequate recanalization, but the outcomes of these specific patients were not reported separately.

Multi-MERCI was a multicenter, prospective, single-arm trial of thrombectomy that included 177 patients with moderate-to-severe large-vessel ischemic strokes [8]. The trial had three broad

aims: (1) to gain greater experience with the first-generation device (X5 and X6) in patients ineligible for IV tPA (patient eligibility in the IV tPA ineligible arm was the same as in the MERCI trial); (2) to explore the safety and technical efficacy data of the device in patients treated with IV tPA who failed to recanalize promptly (patient eligibility in this study arm was the same as those in study arm 1 except that these patients could be enrolled if tPA failed to open the intracranial large vessel as proved by conventional angiography); and (3) to obtain safety and technical data on a second-generation thrombectomy device (L5 Retriever). This device differs from the first generation devices by having a series of monofilaments that attach proximal and distal to the helical nitinol coils. The balloon guide catheter is placed more proximal to arrest flow in the vascular segment as the microcatheter and device are pulled proximally to remove clot. Eligible patients were those within 8 hours of stroke onset who had either failed to respond to intravenous rt-PA or were ineligible for intravenous rt-PA but were still eligible for intra-arterial treatment. The thrombectomy device was deployed successfully in 164 patients. Recanalization was achieved in 55% of patients with the thrombectomy device alone; the percentage of recanalized vessels increased to 68% with combined mechanical and intra-arterial thrombolytic therapy (Table 3.6). Symptomatic intracranial hemorrhage occurred in 9.8% of patients, and significant procedural complications occurred in 5.5% of patients. Good neurological outcomes (modified Rankin scale score ≤2) were observed in 36% of patients at 90 days; however, there was a 34% mortality rate at 90 days. The high mortality may be due to the stroke severity of the cohort (median NIHSS 19 points, interquartile range 15 to 23).

Penumbra system
The FDA approved the Penumbra system in 2007 to open arteries in patients with ischemic strokes. The device is designed to reperfuse large artery occlusions in the intracranial circulation using a suction catheter to aspirate an occlusive thromboembolus while using an internal separator to fragment the clot. A continuous aspiration–debulking process is made possible by advancing and withdrawing the separator through the Penumbra reperfusion catheter into the proximal end of the clot.

The system also contains a thrombus removal ring that can envelop an occlusive clot. If a thrombus remains despite application of the aspiration–debulking components, direct mechanical retrieval by the thrombus removal ring can be used to augment revascularization. Thrombus extraction using the thrombus removal ring is accomplished by engaging the clot proximally and extracting the clot under flow arrest conditions by inflating a proximal balloon guide catheter. Duration of flow arrest is typically less than 1 minute. Patients who have received IV rt-PA can be treated. A video of device deployment can be watched at http://www.youtube.com/watch?v=ajcgsAr6K2A.

Key clinical trials
The Penumbra trial was a prospective, multicenter, single-arm study designed to assess the safety and utility of this device in acute ischemic stroke [9]. Main inclusion and exclusion criteria are listed in Table 3.9. Key clinical inclusion criteria are presentation within 8 hours of symptom onset and a baseline NIHSS of ≥8. Patients treated with intravenous IV r-tPA were eligible if they had persistent neurologic

Table 3.9 Penumbra trial inclusion/exclusion criteria

Inclusion
  Presentation within 8 hours of symptom onset
  NIHSS ≥8
  Angiographically verified occlusion of a large intracranial vessel
  Patients who presented within 3 hours must have been either not eligible or refractory to intravenous recombinant tissue plasminogen activator therapy as defined by the persistence of neurological symptoms and the presence of an occlusion in the target vessel despite the lytic therapy

Exclusion
  Baseline CT showing infarctions greater than one-third of the territory of the middle cerebral artery (MCA), severe edema, or intracranial hemorrhage
  Pregnancy

deficit and angiography demonstrated an occlusion of an appropriate large artery. One hundred twenty-five patients were enrolled at 24 centers. Target arteries were vertebrobasilar (n=11; 9%), middle cerebral (n=87; 70 %), internal carotid (n=23, 18%), and other (n=4; 3%). Twelve of the enrolled patients received intra-arterial thrombolytics (considered a protocol violation) as adjunctive therapy, of which six were targeting the primary obstruction and the remainder aimed at distal branches. Vessel recanalization in those treated with the device alone occurred in nearly 80% of the cases. This recanalization rate is higher than the values observed in the PROACT II, Merci, and Multi-Merci trials (Table 3.6). Twenty-five percent of patients had good neurological outcome, defined as a modified Rankin scale score ≤2 at 3 months following treatment.

Of the 14 symptomatic intracerebral hemorrhages, four were subarachnoid hemorrhages. Six of the patients with symptomatic intracerebral hemorrhage had either intravenous (four patients) or intra-arterial (two patients) fibrinolytic therapy. The authors felt that concomitant use of intravenous or intra-arterial fibrinolytic therapy did not contribute to the rate of intracerebral hemorrhage nor did it seem to be a safety concern when used in conjunction with the Penumbra system. Other adverse procedural events were vasospasm (four), re-occlusion of the target vessel (three), arterial dissection (three), arterial perforation (three), and stroke in a new territory (one).

Solitaire device

In March, 2012 the FDA approved the Solitaire device for mechanical thrombectomy in acute ischemic stroke. The Solitaire device utilizes clot retrieval and suction mechanisms in a sequential fashion. Following microcatheter placement through the clot, the Solitaire device slides through the microcatheter until it also extends through the clot. The microcatheter is then slid back so that the device expands and captures the clot. The Solitaire device is then pulled back and suction is used to remove the clot from the blood vessel. Deployment of this device can be seen at http://www.youtube.com/watch?v=0DQPD5TTS5Y.

FDA approval was based on the Solitaire With the Intention For Thrombectomy (SWIFT) Study. In this randomized study conducted at 18 sites, 113 patients received treatment with either the Solitaire device or the Merci Retriever within 8 hours following stroke onset. The SWIFT study was terminated prematurely because of the effectiveness of the Solitaire Device. Vessel recanalization occurred in 83% treated with Solitaire and 48% who underwent treatment with the Merci Retriever. Mortality at 3 months was lower in the Solitaire arm (17%) than in the Merci arm (38%) and favorable outcome at 3 months was higher in the Solitaire arm (58%) than in the Merci Retriever arm (33%). Study results were presented at the 2012 American Stroke Association International Conference. Study publication is currently pending.

☆ TIPS AND TRICKS

A noninvasive vascular imaging study such as CT angiography or MR angiography may be considered in potential candidates for endovascular reperfusion therapy. This study should include imaging of the extracranial and the intracranial arterial vasculature. Imaging of these vessels can help to define the target vessel for the procedure. In addition, the study can determine if there are radiographic contraindications (e.g. an occluded cervical artery proximal to the occluded intracranial artery, absence of large artery occlusion) to an endovascular procedure.

Postprocedural care

Following an endovascular reperfusion therapy, the patient should be monitored in a critical care setting for approximately 24 hours. Key points regarding care during the first 24 hours following the procedure are similar to those utilized for care of patients treated with intravenous rt-PA:

- Blood pressure monitoring every 15 minutes during the first 2 hours postprocedure, then every 30 minutes for 6 hours, then every 60 minutes for the following 16 hours.
- If systolic blood pressure exceeds 180 mmHg or diastolic blood pressure exceeds 105 mmHg during the post-treatment monitoring period, treat blood pressure with short-acting intravenous antihypertensive drugs such as labetalol (10 mg IV over 1–2 minutes; may repeat every 10–20 minutes with maximal dose 300 mg). If blood pressure fails to respond to adequate doses of labetalol, a continuous antihypertensive infusion should be initiated (labetalol 2–8 mg/minute or nicardipine 5 mg/hour and titrate to goal blood pressure by increasing 2.5 mg/hour every 5 minutes to a maximum dose of 15 mg/hour).
- Obtain noncontrast brain CT at hour 24 +/− 8 hours to evaluate for hemorrhagic trans formation.
- In patients treated with IAT avoid initiation of secondary stroke prevention drug (aspirin, clodipigrel, Aggrenox, intravenous or low-molecular-weight heparin, or warfarin) until the results of the 24 hour CT scan are known and integrated into decision making.
- A secondary preventive agent can be started postprocedurally in patients treated with mechanical embolectomy. Selection of a particular agent is dependent on the presumptive mechanism underlying the ischemic event. Initiation of the secondary preventive drug may be delayed in certain patients, if the treating vascular neurologist and interventionalist feel that early initiation may significantly increase the risk of symptomatic hemorrhagic infarction.
- Avoid subcutaneous heparin or low-molecular-weight heparin for deep venous thrombosis prophylaxis until the results of the 24-hour CT scan are known in IAT-treated patients. Initiation of

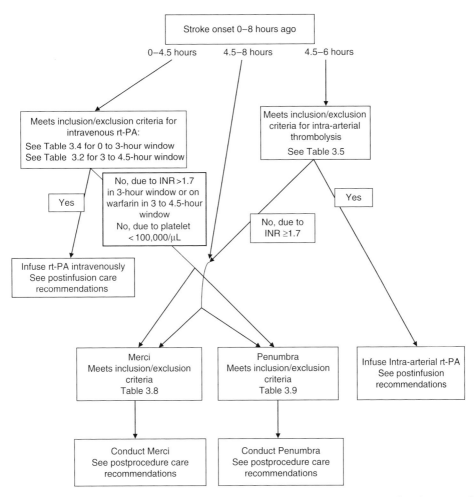

Figure 3.5 Thrombolysis/ mechanical embolectomy decision pathway for patients with ischemic stroke symptoms <8 hours old. Patients who are eligible for intravenous rt-PA and meet criteria for the 3 or 4-hour infusion window should proceed to intravenous rt-PA treatment, rather than being shifted to an intra-arterial procedure. The presence of one of two exclusion criteria for intravenous rt-PA (namely INR ≥1.7 or platelet count <100,000/μL) can exclude a patient from receiving intravenous rt-PA, but the patient may be eligible for treatment with an interventional procedure if the procedure is available. For example a patient with an INR of 1.9 may be treated with Merci in both the 3 and 4.5-hour windows. Likewise, a platelet count of 70,000/μL will prohibit intravenous infusion of rt-PA, but the patient might still meet inclusion criteria for treatment with Merci or Penumbra. The decision to treat a patient within the 4.5 to 6-hour window with intra-arterial rt-PA versus a mechanical procedure is often dependent on the experience of the treating interventionalist. These procedures have not been compared to each other in a clinical trial. Thus, there is no evidence verifying that one of the procedures is better or safer than the other when conducted within this time frame.

subcutaneous heparin or low-molecular-weight heparin does not be need to be delayed in patients who have undergone mechanical thrombectomy.

• Use sequential compression devices for deep venous thrombosis prophylaxis when subcutaneous heparin and low-molecular-weight heparin are contraindicated.

Decision making

The decision to intervene and treat an acute ischemic stroke with intravenous thrombolysis or with an endovascular procedure is determined by obtaining a focused and accurate medical history, determination of NIHSS, review of diagnostic data, discussion with the patient and/or their health-care surrogate, and review with other members of the health-care team. Time of stroke symptom onset is the primary historical point that places a patient on an initial, specific treatment pathway (Figure 3.5). Patients may veer off a treatment path if inclusion criteria are not present or if exclusions to treatment are identified. Patients who present very early following symptom onset should be initially considered for intravenous rt-PA provided the treatment can be administered within the 3 or 4.5-hour window. Patients eligible for intravenous rt-PA should generally not be initially considered for an endovascular therapy as this may introduce unnecessary delays in treatment. In addition, there have not been clinical studies examining the effectiveness of intra-arterial reperfusion procedures versus intravenous thrombolysis in very early stroke. Occasionally, the clinician will care for a patient who does not qualify for intravenous thrombolysis based on the presence of an exclusion criterion. This patient, however, may still be a candidate for IAT (Figure 3.5). If IAT is available, the patient should be evaluated for mechanical thrombectomy.

Future directions

Additional research is needed to discover methods that safely magnify the therapeutic effects of thrombolytic therapy and mechanical thrombectomy. Combining intravenous rt-PA with drugs that are neuroprotectants, drugs that promote collateral blood flow to an ischemic zone, or drugs that are antithrombotic are areas of current investigation. Combining rt-PA and transcranial Doppler ultrasound, so-called sonothrombolysis, is another current avenue of investigation. In the future, well-designed clinical trials may demonstrate that new generation thrombolytic drugs with shorter infusion times and longer half-lives, such as tenecteplase, improve clinical outcomes. Development of appropriate bridging strategies, which utilize upfront treatment with intravenous rt-PA followed by an interventional procedure, is also a subject of ongoing research.

Selected bibliography

1. The National Institute of Neurological Disorders and Stroke rt-PA Stroke Study Group. Tissue plasminogen activator for acute ischemic stroke. *N Engl J Med* 1995; **333**: 1581–7.
2. Hacke W, Kaste M, Bluhmki E, et al. Thrombolysis with alteplase 3 to 4.5 hours after acute ischemic stroke. *N Engl J Med* 2008; **359**: 1317–29.
3. Adams HP Jr, del Zoppo G, Alberts MJ, et al. Guidelines for the early management of adults with ischemic stroke: a guideline from the American Heart Association/American Stroke Association Stroke Council, Clinical Cardiology Council, Cardiovascular Radiology and Intervention Council, and the Atherosclerotic Peripheral Vascular Disease and Quality of Care Outcomes in Research Interdisciplinary Working Groups. *Stroke* 2007; **38**: 1655–711.
4. Furlan A, Higashida R, Weschler L, et al. Intra-arterial prourokinase for acute ischemic stroke. The PROACT II study: a randomized controlled trial. Prolyse in Acute Cerebral Thromboembolism. *JAMA* 1999; **282**: 2003–11.
5. Brandt T, von Kummer R, Müller-Küppers M, Hacke W. Thrombolytic therapy of acute basilar artery occlusion; variables affecting recanalization and outcome. *Stroke* 1996; **27**: 875–81.
6. Jung S, Mono M-L, Fischer U, et al. Three-month and long-term outcomes and their predictors in acute basilar artery occlusion treated with intra-arterial thrombolysis. *Stroke* 2011; **42**: 1946–51.
7. Smith WS, Sung G, Starkman S, et al. Safety and efficacy of mechanical embolectomy in acute ischemic stroke: results of the MERCI Trial. *Stroke* 2005; **36**: 1432–8.
8. Smith WS, Sung G, Saver J, et al. Mechanical thrombectomy for acute ischemic stroke: final results of the Multi Merci trial. *Stroke* 2008; **39**: 1205–39.
9. Penumbra Pivotal Stroke Trial Investigators. The penumbra pivotal stroke trial: safety and effectiveness of a new generation of mechanical devices for clot removal in intracranial large vessel occlusive disease. *Stroke* 2009; **40**: 2761–8.

4

Diagnosis of Stroke Mechanisms and Secondary Prevention

Kelly D. Flemming, MD

Department of Neurology, Mayo Clinic College of Medicine, Rochester, Minnesota

Introduction to diagnostic evaluation

The goal of the diagnostic work up is threefold: (1) to determine a potential mechanism and etiology of cerebral infarction; by doing so, the correct anti-thrombotic (antiplatelet agent versus anticoagulation) can be chosen; (2) to determine and treat contributing risk factors; and (3) to do so in an efficient, cost-effective manner, minimizing harm to the patient.

Cerebral infarction subtype and treatments are diverse. The prevalence of various subtypes differ across age groups, races, and in patients with certain medical conditions. Treatments must weigh the risk and benefit in individuals. Because of all these factors, an algorithmic approach can be complex. However, systematically approaching each patient presenting with a transient neurologic deficit or cerebral infarction can be performed by asking several important questions (Box 4.1). These questions will be expanded upon and a general approach to testing is described in this section.

Do the symptoms represent cerebral ischemia (versus nonischemic pathology)?

When a patient presents with a transient neurologic deficit, one must consider alternative etiologies to transient ischemia [1]. Common mimickers of transient ischemic attack (TIA) and cerebral infarction are noted in Table 4.1. Details from the history and physical examination, as noted above, in addition to imaging studies are useful for distinguishing cerebral ischemia from nonischemic mechanisms.

Where does the process localize?

Three steps are useful when approaching ischemic stroke localization. First, is the ischemic event in the anterior (carotid, middle cerebral artery, anterior cerebral artery) or posterior (vertebrobasilar) circulation (Table 4.2)? This is important if one finds an arterial stenosis to determine whether it is symptomatic or asymptomatic. For instance, management differs significantly when finding a carotid artery stenosis in a patient with an ischemic event in the anterior versus posterior circulation. Second, is the ischemic event cortical or subcortical (Table 4.3)? This is important as cortical events are more likely to be embolic (cardioembolic or artery to artery). Presence of aphasia, cortical sensory loss, or weakness involving predominantly the face and arm greater than the leg (middle cerebral artery) or leg greater than the arm or face (anterior cerebral artery) suggest a cortical deficit. Unilateral face, arm, and leg weakness or numbness equally suggests a subcortical lesion. A third question that may be helpful in determining the mechanism of stroke is whether the stroke involves multiple arterial territories. If so, differential diagnosis includes cardioembolic, coagulation disorder, and multifocal arterial disease (vasculitis, diffuse atherosclerosis, atherosclerosis with congenital anomalies such as a fetal posterior circulation or an absent A1 segment).

After completing the history, physical examination, and initial head CT, one should potentially be able to localize the event to the anterior or

Stroke, First Edition. Edited by Kevin M. Barrett and James F. Meschia.
© 2013 John Wiley & Sons, Ltd. Published 2013 by John Wiley & Sons, Ltd.

> **BOX 4.1 Systematic approach to diagnostic cerebral infarction or TIA evaluation**
>
> 1. Is it an ischemic stroke or TIA (versus nonischemic pathology)?
> 2. Where does the process localize?
> 3. What mechanisms and etiologies are possible?
> 4. What is the prevalence (pretest probability) of each etiology in this patient?
> 5. What treatment is available for this etiology?
> 6. What tests/ studies are useful to evaluate this etiology?

Table 4.1 Mimickers of transient ischemic attack and cerebral infarction

TIA	Cerebral infarction
	Seizure
Seizure	Systemic infection
Migraine equivalent (variant)	Brain tumor
Metabolic	Toxic-metabolic
Multiple sclerosis	Positional vertigo
Myasthenia gravis	Cardiac
Periodic paralysis	Syncope
Thoracic outlet	Trauma
Subdural hemorrhage	Subdural or intracerebral hemorrhage
Transient global amnesia	HSV encephalitis
Reversible vasoconstrictive syndrome	Dementia
	Demyelinating disease
	Myasthenia gravis
	Parkinsonism
SMART syndrome	Hypertensive encephalopathy
	Conversion disorder

Data from Libman R, Wirkowski E, Alvir J, et al. Conditions that mimic stroke in the emergency department. Implications for acute stroke trials. *Arch Neurol* 1995; **52**: 1119–22.

Table 4.2 Anterior versus posterior circulation – symptoms and signs of cerebral ischemia

Anterior circulation	Posterior circulation
Motor dysfunction of contralateral extremities or face (or both): clumsiness weakness paralysis	Motor dysfunction of ipsilateral face and/or contralateral extremities: clumsiness weakness paralysis
Loss of vision in ipsilateral eye	Loss of vision of one or both homonymous visual fields
Homonymous hemianopia	Sensory deficit of ipsilateral face and/or contralateral extremities: numbness or loss of sensation paresthesias
Aphasia (dominant hemisphere)	
Dysarthria	
Sensory deficit of contralateral extremities or face (or both): numbness or loss of sensation paresthesias	Typical, but nondiagnostic in isolation: ataxia (gait or extremities) vertigo diplopia dysphagia dysarthria

Table 4.3 Cortical versus subcortical symptoms and sign of cerebral ischemia

Cortical	Subcortical
Aphasia	Face, arm, and leg more equally affected
Visual field defect	Classic lacunar syndromes:
Monoparesis	pure motor
Hemineglect	pure sensory
Cortical sensory loss	ataxic hemiparesis
Abulia	clumsy-hand dysarthria
	sensorimotor stroke

posterior circulation and have some insight to potential etiologies. If hemorrhage is ruled out and the clinical localization is clear, further imaging such as an MRI is not essential. However, due to transient symptoms, poor description by the patient or witnesses, or symptoms that may localize to either the anterior or posterior circulation, it may not be possible to localize the event clinically. In addition, the initial head CT is often negative, since early infarction signs may not be seen for several hours. In this case, a repeat CT scan after 24 hours of symptoms is a relatively inexpensive way to define the topography of infarction. However, if small vessel disease, brainstem events, or transient symptoms are a concern, an MRI with diffusion weighted images (DWI) would be superior in defining the ischemic site and topography. See also the section below on the utility of cross-sectional imaging.

What are the potential etiologies and mechanisms of cerebral infarction and TIA?

Mechanistically, cerebral ischemia may result from hypoperfusion (low flow), in situ thrombosis, or embolism (cardiac or artery to artery). The actual etiology of these situations may relate to (from proximal to distal): cardioembolic source, large vessel disease of the extracranial vessels (aorta, carotids, vertebrals), large vessel disease of the intracranial vessels, small vessel disease (lacunar), or abnormalities intrinsic to the blood itself, that is coagulation defects (Table 4.4). Despite a thorough diagnostic evaluation, 15–35% of cerebral infarctions remain cryptogenic, that is no definable source [2].

What is the prevalence (pretest probability) of each potential etiology?

What test modalities exist and what is the sensitivity and specificity of such?

The prevalence of a disease and the sensitivity and specificity of a test to find that disease are very important concepts when evaluating cerebral infarction. Recall that prevalence (pretest probability) is the proportion of individuals in a population with a disease at a specific point in time. Sensitivity refers to the proportion of people with disease who have a positive test result and specificity refers to the proportion of people without disease who have a negative test result. Sensitivity and specificity are independent of prevalence. Prevalence does however, effect the positive and negative predictors of a test:

$$Positive\ predictive\ value = Sensitivity \times Prevalence\ / $$
$$(Sensitivity \times Prevalence) + $$
$$(1 - Specificity)(1 - Prevalence)$$

Even if the sensitivity and specificity of a particular diagnostic test are high, the positive predictive value of the test may be poor because of the low prevalence of certain mechanisms of ischemic stroke. For example, intracranial atherosclerosis is responsible for approximately 5–8% of all strokes. The sensitivity and specificity of MR angiography to detect a greater than 50% stenosis of the intracranial arteries is approximately 88% and 96%, respectively. Taking these factors into account, the positive predictive value is 27%. That is, there is a 27%

Table 4.4 Differential diagnosis of cerebral ischemia etiologies

Cardiac
  Atrial fibrillation
  Mitral stenosis
  Left ventricular thrombus
  Atrial myoma
  Dilated cardiomyopathy
  Anterior wall myocardial infarction
  Prosthetic valves
  Endocarditis (bacterial, nonbacterial, marantic)
  Patent foramen ovale
  Atrial septal aneurysm
  Mitral valve calcification
  Fibroelastoma
  Pulmonary fistula (Osler Weber Rendu)
  Air or fat emboli (rare)
Large vessel extracranial
  Atherosclerosis
  Dissection
  Radiation vasculopathy
  Fibromuscular dysplasia
  Vasculitis:
    Takayasu's
    Giant cell arteritis
Large vessel intracranial
  Atherosclerosis
  Dissection
  Inflammatory vasculitis:
    Isolated CNS angiitis
    Necrotizing vasculitides (Wegener's, polyarteritis nodosa, Churg–Strauss, lymphomatoid granulomatosis)
    Hypersensitivity angiitis with connective tissue disease (sarcoid, systemic lupus erythematosus, Sjögren syndrome, rheumatoid arthritis)
    Susac syndrome (retinocochleocerebral arteriopathy)
    Kohlmeier–Degos disease
    Beçhet disease
Infectious vasculitis:
  Varicella zoster virus
  Human immunodeficiency virus
  Hepatitis B and C
  Epstein–Barr virus
  CMV
Noninflammatory vasculopathies:
  Moya Moya
  Drug induced (cocaine, methamphetamine, phenylproponalomaine, ergotamines)
  Radiation induced
  Eales' disease

(Continued)

Table 4.4 (*Cont'd.*)

Arterial dolichoectasia
Endovascular lymphoma
Postpartum cerebral angiopathy
Thrombosed aneurysm with emboli

Small vessel disease
Lipohyalinosis/ atherosclerosis
Vasculitis:
  Varicella zoster vasculitis
  Cryoglobulin-related angiitis
  Angiitis related to lymphatoid
    malignancies
  Henoch-Schönlein purpura
Hematologic and coagulation disorders
Disorders of coagulation factors:
  Protein C or S deficiency
  Antithrombin III deficiency
  Activated protein C resistance/ Factor
    V Leiden mutation
  Prothrombin 20210A mutation
Disorders of red cells:
  Sickle cell anemia
  Polycythemia (primary or secondary)
  Paroxysmal nocturnal hemoglobinuria
Disorders of white cells:
  Lymphoma
  Leukemia
Disorders of platelets:
  Disseminated intravascular
    coagulation (DIC)
  Thrombotic thrombocytopenic purpura
    (TTP)
  Idiopathic thrombocytopenic purpura
  Essential thrombocythemia
  Thrombocytosis
  Paraproteinemia
  Uremia
Disorders of plasma cells:
  Myeloma
  Cryoglobulinemia
Other:
Antiphospholipid antibody syndrome
Hyperhomocysteinemia
Malignancy -associated coagulopathy
Other
Cerebral autosomal dominant arteriopathy
  subcortical infarcts and
  leukoencephalopathy (CADASIL)
Sneddon syndrome
Fabry disease
Mitochondrial encephalopathy lactic acidosis
  and stroke (MELAS)
Homocystinuria
Organic acidemias

probability of true disease if the test is positive. The negative predictive value would be 100%. The value of this test can be improved by selecting patients where the pretest probability is higher than the general population.

It is important to keep in mind that the pretest probability or prevalence of any etiology of cerebral infarction can increase or decrease with the following factors: age greater than versus less than 50 years, race, certain historical or examination findings, and tertiary care versus primary care. The overall prevalence of selected cerebral infarction etiologies in a general population of patients is: cardioembolic (27%), large vessel disease (18%), small vessel disease (17%), other (3%), and cryptogenic (35%) [2].

The prevalences, available diagnostic tests, and their sensitivities and specificities for each specific mechanism are in the section below entitled "Diagnostic evaluation and treatment by etiology."

What are the potential treatment options?

For most mechanisms of cerebral infarction or TIA, antiplatelet agents are indicated. Therefore, diagnostic evaluation is aimed at evaluating potential etiologies that would require something other than an antiplatelet agent, such as surgery, endovascular intervention, anticoagulation, antibiotics, or immunosuppressants (Box 4.2). In addition to discerning the appropriate antithrombotic, careful review and treatment of potential risk factors are important. Treatment recommendations for each mechanism as well as controversies in treatment are elaborated in the section below entitled "Diagnostic evaluation and treatment by etiology."

General approach

As previously mentioned, an algorithmic approach to the diagnostic evaluation of ischemic stroke can be complex due to the potential mechanisms of stroke and the controversies in treatment for some mechanisms. Figure 4.1 displays a general algorithm that can be followed. In addition, Table 4.5 displays tips in the history, physical examination, and/or initial studies that might increase the pretest probability of individual etiologies of cerebral ischemia. In the following section, utility of cross-sectional CT versus MRI will be discussed. In the "Diagnostic evaluation

Box 4.2 Antithrombotic agents and mechanisms of cerebral ischemia

Mechanisms of stroke that antiplatelet agent is recommended
- Small vessel (lacunar) strokes
- Intracranial atherosclerosis with stenosis
- Carotid artery disease (in addition to appropriate intervention)
- Cryptogenic stroke

Mechanisms of stroke that anticoagulation is preferred over antiplatelet agent

- Atrial fibrillation
- Rheumatic mitral disease
- Recent anterior wall MI with LV thrombus
- Phospholipid antibody syndrome

Mechanisms of stroke where controversy exists as to best antithrombotic

- Patent foramen ovale
- Cardiomyopathy
- Isolated spontaneous echo contrast
- Arterial dissection

and treatment by etiology" section you will learn more in detail about the particular source, diagnostic testing, and treatment recommendations in addition to the current American Heart Association class recommendation and level of evidence (Table 4.6). Also, this section will alert you to the controversies that exist due to lack of definitive evidence on treatment. In the final section, two cases help illustrate the overall approach taking into account the six questions discussed above.

The utility of cross-sectional imaging

As previously discussed, a CT scan of the brain is done urgently to help distinguish hemorrhage from ischemia and to potentially identify alternative causes for the patient's symptoms. CT scans are readily available, fast, and well tolerated. However, early ischemia, small vessel infarctions, and more subtle pathologic abnormalities may be missed on CT. MRI with diffusion weighted imaging (DWI) sequences is more sensitive for detecting ischemia,

but is also more expensive, time intensive, and some patients may be intolerant or have devices incompatible with MRI. MRI is not essential in the diagnostic work up of cerebral ischemia, but may provide valuable information (Box 4.3) [3]. For example if a stroke is readily evident on CT, MRI probably does not have a significant added value in most patients. However, when symptoms are transient, the patient's description is poor, the etiology is in question, or the localization and topography (small vessel versus cortical) is in question, MRI can be quite useful. Also, MRI may show silent areas of ischemia in multiple arterial territories in addition to the symptomatic lesion thereby suggesting a proximal etiology. Rarely, DWI is negative in the setting of true cerebral ischemia. This has most often been seen with very small, presumed lacunar infarctions or in cases of oligemia without ischemia in patients scanned very early on after symptoms. There may also be false positives. Those include: demyelinating lesions, some tumors, and herpes encephalitis.

MRI with DWI may be positive in patients with transient symptoms. The longer the symptoms last, the more likely the DWI will be abnormal. This can be useful in confirming the etiology of ischemia, especially in the case of a patient with ambiguous symptoms or poorly described symptoms. In addition, a tissue-based diagnosis of cerebral ischemia has been proposed. Traditionally, a focal neurologic deficit lasting less than 24 hours is considered a TIA. However, it is noted that many of those clinically diagnosed with TIA have true cerebral ischemia documented by DWI. Therefore the new tissue-based definition has been proposed for TIA and stroke. TIA is a transient episode of neurological dysfunction caused by focal brain, spinal cord, or retinal ischemia, without acute infarction [4]. Any patient with a DWI change on MRI would be considered a stroke patient, no matter what the length of symptoms were. Additional studies have shown that patients with transient symptoms with a DWI lesion are more likely to have recurrent stroke in the short term, leading to additional value of MRI in patients with transient symptoms. However, the widespread availability of urgent MR imaging, patients with either intolerances or devices incompatible with MRI, and the cost may limit our ability to clearly define TIA and stroke in this way.

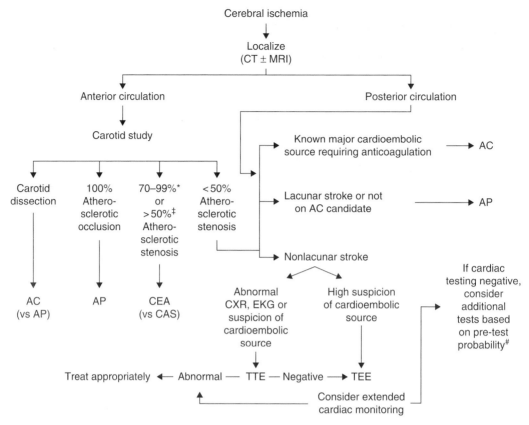

Figure 4.1 General approach to the evaluation of transient ischemic attack and cerebral infarction.
CT, computed tomography; MRI, magnetic resonance imaging;
AC, anticoagulation; AP, antiplatelet agent; CEA, carotid endarterectomy; CAS, carotid angioplasty and stenting; TTE, transthoracic echocardiogram; TEE, transesophageal echocardiogram.
*By noninvasive imaging;
‡by invasive imaging (conventional angiogram);
#see Table 4.5.

Table 4.5 Factors related to the pretest probability of individual stroke mechanisms

Cardioembolic	Large vessel extracranial	Large vessel intracranial	Small vessel	Coagulation
History of atrial fibrillation, congestive heart failure or myocardial infarction	Atherosclerotic risk factors	Atherosclerotic risk factors	Atherosclerotic risk factors	Personal or family history of clotting disorder
Abnormal chest examination	Bruit on examination	Multiple stereotyped transient ischemic attacks	Classic clinical lacunar syndrome	Multiple miscarriages
Abnormal EKG	Systemic symptoms and/ or elevated sedimentation rate (giant cell arteritis)	Systemic symptoms, seizures, young patient (vasculitis)	Waxing/ waning symptoms	Age, race (sickle cell)
Cortical stroke or multiple arterial territories	History of head/ neck injury (dissection)	Illicit drug use		Young age
				Multiple arterial territories
				Venous thrombosis

Table 4.6 Classification of recommendation and level of evidence. From Furie KL, Kasner SE, Adams RJ, et al. Guidelines for the prevention of stroke in patients with stroke or transient ischemic attack: a guideline for healthcare professionals from the American Heart Association/American Stroke Association. *Stroke* 2011; **42**: 227–76.

	SIZE OF TREATMENT EFFECT			
	CLASS I *Benefit >>> Risk* Procedure/Treatment **SHOULD** be performed/administered	**CLASS IIa** *Benefit >> Risk* *Additional studies with focused objectives needed* **IT IS REASONABLE** to perform procedure/administer treatment	**CLASS IIb** *Benefit ≥ Risk* *Additional studies with broad objectives needed; additional registry data would be helpful* Procedure/Treatment **MAY BE CONSIDERED**	**CLASS III** *Risk ≥ Benefit* Procedure/Treatment should **NOT** be performed/administered **SINCE IT IS NOT HELPFUL AND MAY BE HARMFUL**
ESTIMATE OF CERTAINTY (PRECISION) OF TREATMENT EFFECT — **LEVEL A** Multiple populations evaluated* Data derived from multiple randomized clinical trials or meta-analyses	• Recommendation that procedure or treatment is useful/effective • Sufficient evidence from multiple randomized trials or meta-analyses	• Recommendation in favor of treatment or procedure being useful/effective • Some conflicting evidence from multiple randomized trials or meta-analyses	• Recommendation's usefulness/efficacy less well established • Greater conflicting evidence from multiple randomized trials or meta-analyses	• Recommendation that procedure or treatment is not useful/effective and may be harmful • Sufficient evidence from multiple randomized trials or meta-analyses
LEVEL B Limited populations evaluated* Data derived from a single randomized trial or nonrandomized studies	• Recommendation that procedure or treatment is useful/effective • Evidence from single randomized trial or nonrandomized studies	• Recommendation in favor of treatment or procedure being useful/effective • Some conflicting evidence from single randomized trial or nonrandomized studies	• Recommendation's usefulness/efficacy less well established • Greater conflicting evidence from single randomized trial or nonrandomized studies	• Recommendation that procedure or treatment is not useful/effective and may be harmful • Evidence from single randomized trial or nonrandomized studies
LEVEL C Very limited populations evaluated* Only consensus opinion of experts, case studies, or standard of care	• Recommendation that procedure or treatment is useful/effective • Only expert opinion, case studies, or standard of care	• Recommendation in favor of treatment or procedure being useful/effective • Only diverging expert opinion, case studies, standard of care	• Recommendation's usefulness/efficacy less well established • Only diverging expert opinion, case studies, or standard of care	• Recommendation that procedure or treatment is not useful/effective and may be harmful • Only expert opinion, case studies, or standard of care

(Continued)

Table 4.6 (*Cont'd.*)

	SIZE OF TREATMENT EFFECT →		
Suggested phrases for writing recommendations[†]	should is recommended is indicated is useful/effective/ beneficial	is reasonable can be useful/effective/ beneficial is probably recommended or indicated	may/might be considered may/might be reasonable usefulness/effectiveness is unknown/unclear/ uncertain or not well established	is not recommended is not indicated should not is not useful/effective/ beneficial may be harmful

* Data available from clinical trials or registries about the usefulness/efficacy in different subpopulations, such as gender, age, history of diabetes, history of prior myocardial infarction, history of heart failure, and prior aspirin use. A recommendation with Level of Evidence B or C does not imply that the recommendation is weak. Many important clinical questions addressed in the guidelines do not lend themselves to clinical trials. Even though randomized trials are not available, there may be a very clear clinical consensus that a particular test or therapy is useful or effective.

† For recommendations (Class I and IIa; Level of Evidence A and B only) regarding the comparative effectiveness of one treatment with respect to another, these words or phrases may be accompanied by the additional terms "in preference to" or "to choose" to indicate the favored intervention. For example, "Treatment A is recommended in preference to Treatment B for …." or "It is reasonable to choose Treatment A over Treatment B for …." Studies that support the use of comparator verbs should involve direct comparisons of the treatments or strategies being evaluated.

Box 4.3 Advantages of MRI

- Localize cerebral ischemia
- Define topography (cortical versus subcortical)
- Distinguish from nonischemic pathology
- Detect asymptomatic lesions in other territories
- Identify patients with transient symptoms at high risk for recurrence

Box 4.4 Stratifying risk of cerebral ischemia in the setting of atrial fibrillation

CHADS2 score
Congestive heart failure history (1 point)
Hypertension history (1 point)
Age ≥ 75 (1 point)
Diabetes mellitus history (1 point)
Stroke symptoms or TIA (2 points)

Score	Annual stroke risk (%)
0	1.9
1	2.8
2	4.0
3	5.9
4	8.5
5	12.5
6	18.2

Table 4.7 Major versus minor risk cardioembolic sources

Major risk sources	Minor risk sources
Atrial fibrillation	Mitral valve prolapse
Mitral valve stenosis	Severe mitral annular
Prosthetic cardiac valve	calcification
Recent myocardial	Patent foramen ovale
infarction	Atrial septal
Left ventricular or atrial	aneurysm
thrombus	Calcific aortic
Atrial myxoma	stenosis
Infectious endocarditis	Left ventricular
Dilated cardiomyopathy	regional wall motion
Marantic endocarditis	abnormalities
	Mitral valve strands

Diagnostic evaluation and treatment by etiology

Cardioembolic

Prevalence

Approximately 20–30% of cerebral infarctions in a general population have a cardioembolic source. This number does not significantly change with age, however the type of cardioembolic source does. For instance, atrial fibrillation is more common in persons over the age of 75, whereas the potential association of patent foramen ovale and cerebral infarction is more commonly inferred in persons under 50 years of age. In patients with *normal* sinus rhythm, the prevalence of spontaneous echo contrast, left atrial thrombus, and patent foramen ovale (PFO) is 2%, 0.09%, and 25%, respectively.

Sources

Not all cardioembolic sources are of equal risk for future embolic events (Table 4.7). "Major cardiac risk sources" are established as causative risk factors for TIA and cerebral infarction. "Minor risk sources" are established as potential sources and carry an uncertain risk of recurrent stroke due to inconclusive epidemiologic literature.

Atrial fibrillation is a common arrhythmia. It is present in 1% of the general population and up to 10% of those people over the age of 75. Data combined from five primary prevention trials reveal risk factors for ischemic stroke and systemic embolism include: prior stroke or TIA; history of hypertension; congestive heart failure; advanced age; diabetes; coronary artery disease; and left atrial thrombus, spontaneous echo contrast, and left ventricular dysfunction. The risk of stroke may be as high as 10–12% per year with associated risk factors. The CHADS2 (Box 4.4) and CHADS2-VASC scores may help stratify the future risk of cerebral ischemia so this may be weighed against bleeding risks.

One of the more commonly found "minor" sources is the PFO with or without an atrial septal aneurysm. The association of PFO and cerebral infarction has been controversial, with varying results from epidemiologic studies. Most of the studies are case–control design with inherent biases in young patients with cryptogenic stroke. A population-based echocardiographic study suggested a prevalence of 25% in a general population. Risk factors thought to increase the probability that PFO is associated with cerebral infarction include: size, shunting characteristics (right to left), associated atrial septal aneurysm, known deep vein thrombosis, and cortical stroke.

Evaluation

A routine 12-lead electrocardiogram (EKG) is recommended for all patients presenting with cerebral ischemia. In one population-based study, EKG confirmed atrial fibrillation in 25% of patients presenting with first-time stroke. The yield was highest in patients over 80, woman, and those with peripheral vascular and cardiovascular disease.

Paroxysmal atrial fibrillation can be difficult but important to detect. Serial EKGs could be considered and may increase the yield of detection. The yields of 24-hour telemetry and 24 to 48-hour Holter monitoring for detecting paroxysmal atrial fibrillation in unselected patients with cerebral ischemia are approximately 4–8% and 3–5%, respectively [5]. Recently, longer-term heart monitors have proved valuable in the search for patients with paroxysmal atrial fibrillation. Several types of devices exist: patient-triggered event recorder, prolonged ambulatory cardiovascular telemetry, and invasive monitors such as implantable loop recorders and pacemakers [6]. While it is typically not recommended to screen all patients with cerebral ischemia with a Holter monitor or prolonged cardiac monitors, the yield may be increased with certain factors: cortical localization of cerebral ischemia, lack of other cause, enlarged left atrium, mitral valve disease, and older age.

Echocardiography is a useful adjunct to EKG and cardiac monitoring in selected patients with recent cerebral ischemia. Echocardiography may be used to confirm major sources and to detect minor sources of cardioembolism. Transthoracic echocardiogram (TTE) is noninvasive, widely available, and shorter in duration to perform than transesophageal echocardiogram (TEE). TTE can provide a better estimate of left ventricular function and presence of left ventricular thrombus than TEE. However, its use can be limited by the ability to achieve an adequate window in larger patients and its sensitivity in detecting certain embolic sources. TEE is superior in the detection of aortic atheromatous disease or dissection, left atrial thrombus, spontaneous echo contrast (SEC), valvular vegetations, and PFO [5, 7]. Serious complications are rare (<0.02%) when TEE is performed by experienced operators.

A thorough history, physical examination, EKG, and chest X-ray should provide clues to most *major* cardiac sources of embolism. Most minor sources are only detected by TEE, but have no definitive treatment strategies. Therefore, dilemmas arise as to which patients presenting with cerebral infarction or TIA should undergo echocardiography. The yield (or pretest probability) of echocardiography is higher in patients with a history or examination suggestive of cardiac disease, those with a cortical rather than subcortical stroke, and those with an abnormal EKG [5,7]. While the yield may be higher, in some cases it may not change management. For example, a 70-year-old patient with atrial fibrillation may have abnormalities such as spontaneous echo contrast or PFO by echocardiogram, but the patient should be anticoagulated regardless of these findings. In patients without prior history of cardiac disease, the yield is lower, but may be more likely to change management. One study showed that the yield of TEE in patients with large vessel and small vessel disease stroke was only 3%. They also noted that TEE did not change management in those with a known cardioembolic source. Furthermore, in patients with cryptogenic stroke, the yield of TEE was very high and changed management in 30% of cases [8]. Based on this study and others, it is clear that echocardiography in every patient is probably not cost effective, especially for those in whom an alternative mechanism has been found or in whom a known cardioembolic source exists.

Controversy exists on when to do an echocardiogram and by what method. Thus there are few consensus guidelines, but several practical approaches. One older practice guideline suggests: (1) there is fair evidence to recommend echocardiography in patients with stroke and clinical evidence of cardiac disease by history, physical exam, and EKG, or chest X-ray; (2) there is insufficient evidence to recommend for or against TEE in patients with normal TTE; (3) there is insufficient evidence to recommend for or against routine echo in patients, including young patients without clinical cardiac disease; and (4) routine echocardiography is not recommended for patients with clinical cardiac disease who have independent indications for or contraindications to anticoagulant therapy [9]. Another algorithm proposed by Morris and colleagues is presented within the overall algorithm (Figure 4.1) [7].

Other cardiac imaging techniques that may be utilized for detection of thrombus or other structural abnormalities include dual enhanced cardiac CT and cardiac MRI. Dual enhanced cardiac CT is a noninvasive and sensitive way to assess for left atrial spontaneous echo contrast. Cardiac MRI may also be used to help distinguish thrombi from cardiac tumors.

Treatment

Atrial fibrillation: there are class I data that anticoagulation is superior to aspirin and superior to the combination of aspirin and clopidogrel in prevention of cerebral ischemia in patients with atrial fibrillation. Practice guidelines from the American Heart Association recommend: for patients with ischemic stroke or TIA with paroxysmal (intermittent) or permanent AF, anticoagulation with a vitamin K antagonist (target INR 2.5; range 2.0 to 3.0) is recommended (Class I, Level of Evidence A). For patients unable to take oral anticoagulants, aspirin alone (Class I, Level of Evidence A) is recommended [4].

The AHA guidelines were published prior to the FDA approval of dabigatran and rivaroxaban. These anticoagulation alternatives are also options in the prevention of stroke in patients with nonvalvular atrial fibrillation, especially in patients in whom the INR is difficult to manage or are on medications that interact with warfarin.

Other major sources: anticoagulation is preferred over antiplatelet agents for stroke prevention in the setting of prosthetic valves (Class I, Level of Evidence B), rheumatic mitral disease with or without atrial fibrillation (Class IIa, Level of Evidence C), and left ventricular or atrial thrombus. Short-term anticoagulation may be recommended in high-risk patients with a recent myocardial infarction (MI) (Class I, Level of Evidence B). Risk factors include anterior wall MI, coexistence of left ventricular dysfunction or atrial fibrillation, history of hypertension prior to MI, and history of systemic or pulmonary embolism. For patients with ischemic stroke or TIA who have bioprosthetic heart valves with no other source of thromboembolism, anticoagulation with warfarin (INR 2.0 to 3.0) may be considered (Class IIb, Level of Evidence C). Antiplatelet agents are recommended for secondary stroke prevention in those with native aortic or nonrheumatic mitral disease (Class IIb, Level of Evidence C). No firm consensus has been reached regarding an antiplatelet agent versus anticoagulant in cardiomyopathy (ejection fraction (EF) <35%). Infectious endocarditis is treated with antibiotics.

Patent foramen ovale (PFO)/ atrial septal aneurysm: treatment of this entity is controversial. In a prospective, multicenter observational study, 581 patients between 18 and 55 years with cryptogenic ischemic stroke were all placed on aspirin. After 4 years, the recurrent stroke risk was 2.3% among patients with PFO alone, 15.2% in patients with PFO and atrial septal aneurysms, and 4.2% in patients with neither abnormality [10]. This suggests that there may be a population of stroke patients with PFO at higher risk than others and may require treatment other than an antiplatelet agent. However, other studies have suggested no relationship of PFO and ischemic stroke. Options include antiplatelet agents, anticoagulation, closure of the PFO with an endovascular device, or open heart surgery and repair of the PFO. There is no definitive data on which treatment is better than aspirin and each has its own associated risks. Studies on both device closure and surgery suggest a recurrent stroke risk of 3–4% per year. The latter suggests other mechanisms may be playing a role. The AHA recommends that patients with an ischemic stroke or TIA and a PFO, antiplatelet therapy is reasonable (Class IIa, Level of Evidence B) [4].

Other minor sources: no definitive evidence exists for the treatment mitral valve strands, mitral annular calcification, and mitral valve prolapse. In the setting of cerebral ischemia, antiplatelet agent is recommended if these entities are found (Class IIb, Level of Evidence C).

Recommendation

All patients should undergo a clinical evaluation, standard 12-lead EKG, cardiac enzymes, and chest X-ray.

- It is recommended that all patients undergo at least 24 hours of telemetry during a hospital admission for cerebral ischemia.
- Holter monitor and prolonged cardiac monitors are not necessary in every patient. However in

cases of suspected paroxysmal atrial fibrillation, these may prove to be of higher value. Risk factors for paroxysmal atrial fibrillation include: enlarged left atrium, spontaneous echo contrast, cortical ischemic stroke, multiple vascular territory cerebral ischemia, cryptogenic stroke, age, and high frequency of atrial ectopy.

- Echocardiography is not indicated in patients who are clearly not anticoagulation candidates and endocarditis is not a consideration or in patients in whom anticoagulation is required for another reason. If an EKG reveals evidence of atrial fibrillation, an echocardiogram is not indicated unless there is suspicion of endocarditis or the patient is undergoing elective cardioversion.
- Echocardiography should be performed in patients with history (ischemic events in multiple territories), examination (murmur), or routine studies (EKG, cardiac enzymes) suggestive of cardiac disease. In addition, echocardiography could be considered in young patients with cryptogenic stroke and patients with cortical TIA or cerebral infarction, when noninvasive arterial studies are negative. As new studies determine the best treatments for aortic atheromatous disease, PFO, and atrial septal aneurysm, indications for performing echocardiography may be more clearly defined.
- Blood cultures or antinuclear antibody testing should be pursued if bacterial or nonbacterial endocarditis is a clinical consideration.

Large vessel extracranial

Prevalence

Approximately 15–20% of strokes are secondary to large vessel disease (Petty, Brown et al. 1999). Data suggests more than 75% of large vessel disease is due to extracranial disease, that is the extracranial portion of the carotid artery, the vertebral artery, or the aorta. The probability of extracranial large vessel disease due to atherosclerosis increases with typical atherosclerotic risk factors such as hypertension, hyperlipidemia, diabetes, and smoking. The probability of dissection increases with a history of associated neck trauma and pain as well as younger age.

Sources

Extracranial carotid or vertebral disease is most commonly due to atherosclerosis, but can also be due to arterial dissection, Takayasu's arteritis, Giant cell arteritis, radiation, and fibromuscular dysplasia.

Aortic atherosclerotic disease may be a potential source for cerebral infarction. Epidemiologic data suggests that greater than or equal to 4 mm aortic plaque may be an independent risk for stroke.

Evaluation

The goal of evaluating the arterial circulation is to evaluate for evidence and degree of arterial stenosis, determine the location and potential etiology (that is atherosclerosis versus dissection), and to identify other vascular lesions. The choice of diagnostic study to evaluate the extracranial arteries depends on clinical suspicion of etiology, that is atherosclerosis, arteritis, dissection, or other causes.

Carotid ultrasound: an ultrasound is relatively inexpensive, noninvasive, with high sensitivity and specificity for detecting stenosis at the bifurcation. The sensitivity and specificity of color-flow duplex carotid ultrasound to detect internal carotid artery stenosis greater than 70% ranges from 87–95% and 86–97%, respectively [11,12,13]. False-positive carotid ultrasound readings of total carotid occlusion, when there is near total occlusion by arteriography, can occur in 2–7.5%, suggesting a confirmatory test may be required [14, 15].

The main limitation of carotid ultrasound is that it is highly operator dependent. In addition, if the contralateral internal carotid artery is occluded, there can be increased flow on the opposite side that may overestimate the degree of stenosis. For pathologies such as fibromuscular dysplasia, arteritis, or dissection, magnetic resonance angiography (MRA), computed tomography angiography (CTA), or conventional angiography may be superior.

Computed tomography angiography (CTA): CTA is a noninvasive study to evaluate either extracranial or intracranial cerebral circulation. The sensitivity and specificity of CTA to determine an internal carotid artery stenosis greater than 70% is 74–100% and 83–100%, respectively. Sensitivity for detecting carotid artery occlusion is 100%. Unlike MRA, CTA may aid surgeons in localizing bony landmarks as well [16].

The main limitations of CTA are conditions that would not allow contrast dye, such as renal failure and allergy to contrast dye. In addition, if the carotid bifurcation is highly calcified, there may be limitations in determining the exact degree of stenosis. Metallic objects such as clips may also limit view of the artery.

Magnetic resonance angiography (MRA): MRA has evolved significantly over the last 10–15 years with improving sensitivity and specificity to define stenosis and types of pathology. MRA has a sensitivity 83–95% and specificity of 89–94% for the detection of an extracranial internal carotid artery bifurcation stenosis of greater than 70% [13]. The sensitivities and specificities are similar in order to detect a stenosis of greater than 50%. For occlusion, the sensitivity and specificity were 98% and 100%, respectively. MRA technique influences the sensitivity and specificity significantly.

The main limitations of MRA are the cost and availability of the technique. Some methods can overestimate the degree of stenosis with concurrence rates with angiography ranging from 39–98% depending on the technique. Subtle pathology can be missed, such as fibromuscular dysplasia or arteritis. As with any type of MR imaging, the study is contraindicated in patients with ferromagnetic devices, including pacemakers, and gadolinium-enhanced MRA is contraindicated in those with several renal impairment due to nephrogenic systemic fibrosis.

Arteriography: conventional arteriography is considered the gold standard of assessment of the cerebral vasculature. In regards to the extracranial circulation, it is the standard for assessment of degree of internal carotid artery stenosis and is better for detecting plaque morphology, evidence of dissection, and fibromuscular dysplasia than standard MRA or CTA. Furthermore, it can be helpful as a confirmatory test to carotid ultrasound for complete carotid occlusion. A diagnostic arteriography is commonly done prior to carotid artery angioplasty and stenting to confirm the degree of stenosis prior to the procedure and is also used when noninvasive tests show disparate results. The main limitations are the additional cost and risk of the study. There is a 0.5–1% risk of cerebral infarction, TIA, or hematoma formation during the procedure. In addition, renal failure and contrast allergies are relative contraindications.

Transesophageal echocardiography (TEE): TEE is superior to MRA of the aortic arch for detection and quantification of aortic plaque.

Treatment

Symptomatic internal carotid artery stenosis: when cerebral infarction or TIA symptoms are in the anterior circulation ipsilateral to the atheromatous stenotic carotid artery, there is Class I evidence favoring carotid intervention in patients with stenosis greater than or equal to 70% by noninvasive imaging (Level of Evidence A) or 50% or greater by conventional angiography (Level of Evidence B) in whom the risk of intervention is anticipated to be <6% [16]. This should be done ideally within 2 weeks of the incident event [16].

Data from the Northern American Symptomatic Carotid Endarterectomy Trial (NASCET) showed an absolute risk reduction of 17% over 2 years in those surgically treated versus medically treated. The 2-year ipsilateral stroke rate was 26% in the medically treated versus 9% in the carotid endarterectomy (CEA) group [17]. In a NASCET substudy, patients with symptomatic carotid artery disease 50–69% had a 5-year risk of fatal or nonfatal ipsilateral stroke of 22% in the medical group and 15.7% in the surgical group. The long-term benefit of surgery was greater and the risk of stroke with medical treatment was higher for men than for women, for patients who have had stroke than for those with transient ischemic attacks, and for patients with hemispheric symptoms than for those with retinal symptoms. It was also noted that the risk of perioperative stroke or death increased in patients with diabetes, elevated blood pressure, contralateral occlusion, or left-sided disease. There was no evidence for the benefit of CEA for less than 50% stenosis or complete occlusion.

An alternative to CEA is carotid angioplasty and stenting (CAS). Several important clinical trials evaluating the utility of CEA versus CAS in symptomatic patients deserve attention. A number of early studies failed to show that CAS was superior to CEA, but had many study design issues and enrollment issues [16]. The SAPPHIRE trial compared CAS to CEA in both symptomatic and asymptomatic patients considered at high risk for surgery. In this randomized noninferiority trial, the adverse event rate in the CAS group was approximately 6%⁰ and was significantly lower than that of the CEA group. The relatively high adverse event rate in the CEA arm was not unexpected, since these patients were considered at high risk for CEA. The occurrence of the primary endpoint was similar in both groups for symptomatic patients. SAPPHIRE concluded that CAS was not inferior to CEA in patients at high risk for surgery. The SAPPHIRE trial utilized a distal protection device and was carried out by highly experienced operators.

The International Carotid Stenting Study (ICSS) compared the safety and efficacy of CEA to CAS in symptomatic patients with 50% or greater ipsilateral carotid stenosis. The 120-day follow-up rate of stroke, death, or procedural MI was 8.5% in the CAS group versus 5.2% in the CEA group. Longer-term follow-up of this cohort is pending [18].

CREST (Carotid Revascularization Endarterectomy versus Stent Trial) was a randomized trial comparing CAS with CEA in both asymptomatic and symptomatic patients. For the combined endpoint of stroke, death, or MI there was no significant difference in primary events. Stroke was more frequent with CAS, and MI more frequent with CEA [19].

Current American Heart Association Guidelines recommend CAS to be considered in symptomatic patients at average or low risk of complications associated with endovascular intervention (Class I, Level of Evidence B) [4,16]. For patients considered high risk for CEA, CAS may be preferred. These high-risk patients may include: clinically significant cardiac disease, significant pulmonary disease, contralateral carotid occlusion, contralateral laryngeal nerve palsy, previous radical neck surgery or radiation to the neck, and recurrent stenonsis after CEA.

Medically, antiplatelet agents are recommended postendarterectomy or CAS. In addition, a statin would be indicated as well as other assessment of atherosclerotic vascular risk factors.

Internal carotid artery occlusion: symptomatic internal artery occlusion may be responsible for 10–15% of large artery cerebral infarctions. The best medical management (anticoagulation versus antiplatelet therapy) and best surgical management remain to be defined. Some propose using short-term anticoagulation with acute symptomatic occlusion to prevent so-called stump emboli; however, this has not been proven by clinical trial data. Extracranial to intracranial bypass (EC-IC) was routine prior to a 1985 publication reporting that bypass was not helpful in reducing future cerebral infarction in patients with either complete internal carotid artery occlusion, intracranial internal carotid artery stenosis, or middle cerebral artery stenosis.

At this point in time, antiplatelet agent and risk factor management as well as avoiding hypotension are recommended.

EVIDENCE AT A GLANCE

The Carotid Occlusion Surgery Study (COSS) study used oxygen extraction positron emission tomography (PET) scanning to identify patients at high risk for recurrent stroke and randomized them to EC-IC bypass versus medical management [20]. In this study, patients in the surgical arm again had higher rates of early stroke compared to medical management; however, patients were randomized an average of 72 days after incident event. In very select patients failing medical management EC-IC bypass may be considered but this is of unclear value.

Extracranial vertebral artery atherosclerosis: the prevalence of symptomatic vertebral artery stenosis due to atherosclerosis has not been well studied, but may account for 10–20% of patients with posterior circulation cerebral ischemia. Atherosclerosis of the vertebral artery most commonly affects the origin or the vertebrobasilar junction. The AHA recommends consideration of CTA or MRA as part of the initial evaluation of patients with neurologic symptoms referable to the posterior circulation and those with subclavian steal syndrome (Class I, Level of Evidence C) [16]. It is this author's opinion that since first-line treatment for vertebral artery stenosis is antiplatelet agent, imaging in all patients with posterior circulation events is not cost effective or necessary. For those patients with an alternative source already determined (example: cardioembolic source) or those not currently on antiplatelet agents, imaging may not change management and is therefore not necessarily warranted. However, in patients in whom no alternative cause is noted and have already been on antiplatelet agent, imaging may prove more valuable. If it is found to be the cause of cerebral ischemia, antiplatelet agent and vascular risk factor management is first-line treatment. In cases of medical "failure" with recurrent cerebral ischemic events, angioplasty and stenting is a consideration.

Subclavian and innominate atherosclerosis: subclavian stenosis and innominate artery atherosclerosis is a rare cause of cerebral ischemia, but should be considered in patients with symptoms of cerebral ischemia and arm or hand claudication. Extra anatomic carotid–subclavian bypass or endovascular angioplasty and stenting can be considered in patients with severe subclavian disease resulting in cerebral ischemia (Class IIa, Level of Evidence C). Arterial reconstruction, extra-anatomic bypass surgery, or angioplasty and stenting is considered in patients with symptomatic innominate artery stenosis (Class IIa, Level of Evidence C).

Carotid or vertebral dissection: MRA, CTA, or conventional angiography are superior to ultrasound for detection of extracranial artery dissection of the carotid or vertebral arteries (Class I, Level of Evidence C). The American Heart Association Guidelines suggests that for patients with ischemic stroke or TIA and extracranial carotid or vertebral arterial dissection, antithrombotic treatment for at least 3 to 6 months is reasonable (Class IIa, Level of Evidence B) [4]. However, there are no randomized clinical trial data to address the question of whether anticoagulation is better than antiplatelet agents in cervical arterial dissection. While many clinicians will anticoagulate patients with arterial dissection for a period of 3 to 6 months, then switch to an antiplatelet agent, this is based on expert opinion. If a patient fails medical therapy, endovascular stenting or surgery can be considered.

Aortic atherosclerosis: a retrospective study found that anticoagulation was better than antiplatelet agents in patients with aortic atheroma >4 mm with or without debris. Those on antiplatelet had a 5.9 times chance of recurrent events, although the confidence intervals were wide.

> **EVIDENCE AT A GLANCE**
>
> The Warfarin–Aspirin Recurrent Stroke Study Group (WARRS) attempted to determine if warfarin is effective and superior to aspirin in prevention of noncardioembolic ischemic stroke. Patients were randomized to either warfarin (goal INR 1.4–2.8) versus aspirin (325 mg/day). The primary endpoint was recurrent ischemic stroke or death from any cause within 2 years. There was no difference in primary outcomes over 2 years. This trial included patients with aortic atherosclerosis, although it was only a small subgroup [21].

An ongoing study, ARCH (Aortic Arch Related Cerebral Hazard Trial), is randomizing patients to warfarin (goal INR 2–3) versus aspirin and clopidogrel in patients with aortic arch atherosclerosis and recent stroke or peripheral emboli. Therefore, at this time, best antithrombotic management is not defined. In general, however, if mobile debris is associated with the aortic plaque, anticoagulation is often used over an antiplatelet agent. However if there is no associated mobile debris, an antiplatelet agent and statin are favored.

Recommendation

• If a patient has a cerebral infarction or TIA referable to the anterior circulation, the extracranial carotid arteries need to be assessed since definitive evidence for treatment of carotid artery stenosis due to atherosclerosis exists. Be aware of the occasional congenital anomalies such as the fetal posterior cerebral artery when evaluating a patient with high-grade atherosclerosis of the bifurcaton.

• The choice of tests may reflect the expected etiology. For instance, if dissection is a concern, MRA or CTA may be considered first. If the patient is over 55 years and has typical atherosclerotic risk factors, a carotid ultrasound could be considered first. If carotid atherosclerosis is noted by ultrasound, a second noninvasive imaging study may be warranted for confirmation and to assess anatomic considerations for surgery, including collateral circulation.

- If the patient has symptoms localizing to the posterior circulation, MRA or CTA of the neck could be considered, especially if dissection is a consideration or if the patient has failed antiplatelet therapy and no other source of cerebral ischemia has been found.
- Evaluation for aortic atherosclerosis can be performed with TEE. However, since definitive management for this entity is unknown, this is not an essential diagnosis to make currently. One might consider evaluating for this if the patient has multiple arterial territory infarctions, a history of peripheral vascular disease, or has "failed" antiplatelet therapy.

Large vessel intracranial

Prevalence

Epidemiologic studies suggest that 5–8% of strokes are due to large vessel intracranial disease. The pretest probability increases in women, Asian, African, or Hispanic Americans, diabetics, patients with cortical symptoms or recurrent stereotyped TIAs in a single vascular territory, and posterior circulation events.

Sources

Intracranial disease may be due to atherosclerosis, dissection, vasculitis, noninflammatory vasculopathy, Moya Moya disease, radiation changes, thrombosed aneurysm with distal emboli, and vasospasm (reversible cerebrovasoconstrictive syndrome).

Evaluation

Options for the evaluation of intracranial disease include: MR angiography, CT angiography, transcranial Doppler, and conventional arteriography.

Transcranial Doppler (TCD): transcranial Doppler ultrasound is a noninvasive technique to assess the proximal intracranial internal carotid artery, the M-1 segment of the middle cerebral artery, the A-1 segment of the anterior cerebral artery, the vertebral arteries, and the proximal aspect of the basilar artery. For all vessels, TCD has a sensitivity of 89–98%, and a specificity of 87–96% for detecting stenosis greater than 50%. Sensitivity for detection of occlusion varies by site: proximal internal carotid artery 94%, distal internal carotid artery 81%, middle cerebral artery 93%, terminal vertebral artery 56%, and basilar artery 60%. Specificity for occlusion ranges from 96 to 98% [22].

> ✋ **CAUTION**
>
> Transcranial Dopper is highly operator dependent and the transtemporal window may not allow insonation of the proximal middle cerebral artery, anterior cerebral artery, or posterior cerebral artery in up to 20% of patients.

CTA: few data exist regarding the sensitivity and specificity of CTA in detection of intracranial disease. Skutta and colleagues report the sensitivity of double-detector helical CT angiography in the detection of intracranial stenosis as compared to conventional arteriography. The sensitivity was 61% for detection of 30–69% stenosis, 78% for detection of 70–99% stenosis, and 100% for occluded segments [23]. Concurrence with conventional arteriography was best in the basilar artery (92%) and the A-2 segment (100%). Concurrence for other intracranial segments ranged from 45–85%. As with any new study, evolving technology will likely improve on this sensitivity over time. The main limitation of CT angiography, as previously noted, is the use of contrast dye.

MRA: MR angiography has the advantage over CT angiography of not requiring iodinated contrast dye. The main limitation, as with any MR study, is that it is contraindicated in patients with ferromagnetic devices. The sensitivity and specificity of three-dimensional time-of-flight angiography to detect stenoses greater than 50% approximately ranges in the literature from 85–88% and 96–97%, respectively [22]. Technologies are evolving, including the use of gadolinium bolus intracranial MRA, which will likely improve on these data in time.

Arteriogram: conventional arteriography is the gold standard for detecting the degree of arterial stenosis and is superior to noninvasive studies for evaluating arteries distal to the circle of Willis, such as those often involved in vasculitis. It is also superior in detecting arteriovenous malformations or dural arteriovenous fistulas, which may also present with transient neurologic deficits, and in defining plaque and vessel pathology. Other indications may include equivocal or conflicting noninvasive studies. The limitations of this test are noted in the previous section.

Treatment

A subgroup analysis of the WARRS trial included "large artery stenosis or occlusion." This group comprised 10% of the study population and reflected extracranial carotid artery occlusion as well as intracranial stenosis. There was no difference in patients randomized to warfarin (INR 1.4–2.8) or aspirin (325 mg/day) [21].

Based on a retrospective study favoring warfarin over antiplatelet agent in symptomatic intracranial stenosis, WASID (Warfarin and Aspirin for Symptomatic Intracranial Disease) investigators prospectively randomized patients to warfarin (INR goal 2–3) versus aspirin (1300 mg/day). The trial was stopped early due to excess mortality of those patients receiving warfarin. After 1.8 years, the primary endpoint of ischemic stroke, brain hemorrhage, or death from vascular cause was reached in 22.1% of patients in the aspirin group and 21.8% of patients in the warfarin group [24].

EVIDENCE AT A GLANCE

The SAMMPRIS (Stenting and Aggressive Medical Management for Preventing Recurrent Stroke in Intracranial Stenosis) trial randomized patients with cerebral ischemia and intracranial arterial stenosis of 70–99% to medical management versus medical management and angioplasty and stenting using the Wingspan stent system. Medical management included aspirin 325 mg daily, clopidogrel 75 mg daily for 90 days, in addition to low-density lipoprotein (LDL) goal <70 mg/dL and aggressive management of blood pressure and other vascular risk factors. The primary endpoint of stroke or death within 30 days was higher in the angioplasty and stent group than medical management (14.7% versus 5.8%) [25].

Bypass procedures for the anterior and posterior circulation exist; however, for intracranial stenosis, there is no current proven benefit based on the Extracranial-Intracranial Bypass Trial and the COSS study [20].

Thus the trials have lead to the American Heart Association recommending antiplatelet therapy and risk-factor management for patients with intracranial stenosis due to atherosclerosis [4,26].

As with any atherosclerotic vascular disease, vascular risk factors should be assessed and treated. However, optimal blood pressure in the setting of a fixed intracranial stenosis is not well defined.

Recommendation

- Evaluation of the *extra*cranial arteries would be recommended first as the pretest probability of extracranial disease is generally higher in both young and older patients.
- Similarly, the pretest probability of a cardio-embolic source may be higher and consideration of echocardiogram should be made on an individual basis (see cardioembolic section above). This is important since most forms of extracranial disease and cardioembolic sources have definitive management strategies.
- After more common entities have been eliminated as sources, evaluation of the intracranial circulation may be recommended in the following patients or situations where the prevalence may be higher: (1) young patient (less than 50 years old) with negative *extra*cranial evaluation and cardiac evaluation; (2) patient has failed antiplatelet therapy and may have recurrent stereotyped TIAs or *cortical* stroke in a single vascular territory; (3) posterior circulation event with negative cardiac evaluation; and (4) preoperative evaluation of collateral circulation prior to carotid endarterectomy.

Small vessel disease

Prevalence

Small vessel (lacunar) infarctions account for up to 20% of all cerebral ischemic events. Since lacunar infarctions are associated microscopically with microatheroma, lipohyalinosis, and fibrinoid necrosis, the pretest probability increases with typical atherosclerotic risk factors, most notably hypertension, smoking, and diabetes.

Sources

A lacunar stroke is a small subcortical infarction generally defined as a stroke less than 1.5 cm resulting from the occlusion of a penetrating end artery. Penetrating end arteries may include:

Table 4.8 Lacunar syndromes

Lacunar syndrome	Localization
Pure motor hemiparesis	Posterior internal capsule, corona radiata
Pure sensory stroke	Thalamus
Ataxic hemiparesis	Pons, posterior internal capsule/ corona radiata
Clumsy hand-dysarthria	Pons
Sensorimotor stroke	Posterior internal capsule and thalamus

lenticulostriates, thalamoperforates, basilar artery perforates, and others. Thus lacunes predominate in the basal ganglia, thalamus, centrum semiovale, brain stem, and internal capsule. Typical lacunar clinical syndromes and common anatomic locations are noted in Table 4.8. Autopsy studies have shown that the pathology underlying lacunar infarctions is most commonly microatheroma, lipohyalinosis, and fibrinoid necrosis. However, in approximately 5–10% of autopsy cases these findings are not seen, implying the possibility that lacunar infarctions could result from an embolic source. While some believe that carotid imaging is not necessary in classic cases of lacunar disease, the NASCET study evaluating the efficacy of carotid endarterectomy for carotid stenosis as well as the CREST study did consider patients with lacunar infarctions and ipsilateral carotid disease as symptomatic.

Other etiologies of stroke may result in small vessel pathology. These include: certain coagulation disorders, small vessel vasculitides (Behçet's, cryoglobulin-related angiitis, angiitis related to lymphatoid malignancies, varicella zoster vasculitis), and Henoch–Schönlein purpura.

Evaluation

Since lipohyalinosis and microatheroma are not visible by any diagnostic techniques, the clinical onset, patient risk factors, examination, and topography of the infarction become important. The lacunar hypothesis states that patients present with a small number of distinct lacunar syndromes, and secondly that lacunes are caused by characteristic disease of the penetrating endartery. Gan and colleagues, examined 591 patients to determine the value of the clinical lacunar

syndrome in predicting radiologic lacunes and the value of clinicoradiologic lacunes in predicting lacunar infarction as the final stroke mechanism [27]. The clinical lacunar syndromes of pure sensory stroke, ataxic hemiparesis, sensorimotor stroke, and pure motor hemiparesis had positive predictive values of 100%, 95%, 87%, and 79%, respectively, of detecting a radiographic lacune. The final mechanism in persons presenting with a lacunar syndrome and radiographic evidence of lacune were: 75% small vessel disease, 9% atherosclerosis, 5% cardioembolic, 9% cryptogenic, and 2% unusual. Thus, authors concluded that while pure sensory stroke and ataxic hemiparesis presentations were highly predictive of a small vessel disease, 25% of persons presenting with a clinical lacunar syndrome confirmed radiographically could have other potential mechanisms, warranting alternative treatment.

Treatment

For common lacunar infarction presumed due to lipohyalinosis, antiplatelet agents and aggressive risk factor management are warranted, unless other mechanisms are found.

Recommendation

- Consider MRI in patients in the setting of a lacunar syndrome to confirm topography since clinical localization is not completely accurate other than for pure sensory stroke.
- A study of the extracranial carotid artery is recommended in patients with lacunar infarctions in the anterior circulation.
- Further noninvasive diagnostic studies appropriate to the potential localization of the infarct (see other sections) may be warranted if:

1) patient lacks typical atherosclerotic risk factors;
2) presents with an atypical clinical lacunar syndrome;
3) there is radiographic evidence of a lacune in an atypical territory;
4) has a typical lacunar clinical syndrome but imaging reveals a cortical infarction.

Coagulation disorders

Prevalence

The prevalence of specific coagulation disorders in the general population are noted in Table 4.9. As a

Table 4.9 Prevalence of coagulation abnormalities in the general population

Factor	Prevalence in population
Antiphospholipid antibody	2–5%
Factor V Leiden factor/ Activated protein C resistance	1–9%
Congenital protein C deficiency	1 in 36,000
Congenital protein S deficiency	1 in 15,000–20,000
Congenital antithrombin III deficiency	1 in 2000–5000
Homocysteine (moderate)	30% of stroke population

cause for stroke, coagulation disorders account for 1–4.8% of all strokes. The pretest probability, or prevalence, of these entities increases in younger patients (under 45 years), patients with prior history of clotting dysfunction, and in patients with cryptogenic stroke.

Sources

The following abnormalities have been associated with arterial cerebral infarction: sickle cell anemia, polycythemia vera, essential thrombocythemia, heparin-induced thrombocytopenia, disseminated intravascular coagulopathy, thrombocytosis, protein C or S deficiency (acquired or congenital), antithrombin III deficiency, antiphospholipid antibody syndrome, and hyperhomocysteinemia. Factor V Leiden mutation and prothrombin 20210 mutations predispose to venous thrombosis. They may result in cerebral venous thrombosis or possibly be associated with deep venous thrombosis with paradoxical emboli.

Evaluation

All patients should have a CBC, aPTT, INR, and sedimentation rate. Selected patients may require additional testing including: homocysteine, coagulation factors, disseminated intravascular coagulation (DIC) panel, Factor V and Prothrombin 20210 mutations, antiphospholipid antibodies and lupus anticoagulant testing, and hemoglobin electrophoresis.

Treatment

In patients with cryptogenic cerebral ischemia in whom an antiphospholipid antibody is detected, an antiplatelet agent is recommended (Class IIa, Level of Evidence B). This recommendation is based on a small subgroup analysis of the WARRS trial, which suggested no difference in outcome with aspirin versus warfarin (INR 1.4–2.8) in patients with a detected phospholipid antibody. However, in those patients with cryptogenic cerebral ischemia meeting the criteria for phospholipid antibody syndrome, anticoagulation with a goal INR of 2–3 is recommended (Class IIa, Level of Evidence B).

Elevated homocysteine can be treated with supplemental B12, B6, and folate. Studies show that the homocysteine level responds to treatment; however, no study to date shows reduction in recurrent stroke because of treatment in patients with mild to moderate elevations of homocysteine and cerebral ischemia.

Primary prevention trials for sickle cell anemia have shown benefit with transfusion therapy (STOP trial). However, there are no randomized secondary prevention trials. Limited retrospective data with secondary prevention is largely based on studies of children, and so recommendations for adults lack significant evidence. Thus, therapies that may be considered to prevent recurrent cerebral ischemic events in patients with sickle cell disease (SCD) include regular blood transfusions to reduce hemoglobin S to 30–50% of total hemoglobin, hydroxyurea, or bypass surgery in cases of advanced occlusive disease (Class IIb, Level of Evidence C).

Recommendation

- All patients should have a CBC, aPTT, INR, and sedimentation rate.
- Patients with a high pretest probability for a coagulation disorder should undergo additional coagulation studies. Pretest probability increases with: patients under 45 years with no other source determined, patients with personal or family history of clotting disorders, or venous infarction.

Risk factors

A diagnostic evaluation is not complete without further evaluating cerebrovascular risk factors. This should include a fasting lipid screen, fasting glucose, and assessment of blood pressure, body mass index, diet, exercise, questions regarding sleep apnea symptoms, and tobacco and alcohol use. One may also consider screening for medical complications related to cerebral ischemia including: depression, venous thromboembolism risk, aspiration risk, fall risk, and gastrointestinal bleed risk.

Case examples

CASE 1

A 72-year-old Caucasian man with a history of hyperlipidemia and hypertension who presents with a 5-minute spell of right face and arm heaviness. An hour later he had another spell of right face and arm heaviness, this time accompanied by difficulty getting words out. This lasted approximately 5 minutes and resolved. The patient was taken to the emergency room where initial head CT, EKG, and laboratory studies are normal.

Answering the questions

1) **Is it an ischemic event?**
   The patient's symptoms came on acutely and are in a vascular territory. He is of a common age and gender with vascular risk factors for cerebral ischemia. Therefore one would consider this a probable ischemic vascular event.
2) **Where does the process localize?**
   Right face and arm heaviness or weakness should localize to the left hemisphere in the anterior circulation (carotid distribution). Since it is face and arm more than leg, it may be more cortical than subcortical. Furthermore the word-finding difficulty may suggest cortical involvement as well, that is aphasia.
3) **What mechanisms and etiologies are possible?**
   The past medical history of hypertension and hyperlipidemia are risk factors for atherosclerotic disease. The fact that patient has had three stereotyped spells in one vascular territory suggest a possible focal arterial stenosis. In this man, extracranial internal carotid artery stenosis is most likely given the higher prevalence of extracranial carotid disease in Caucasians compared to intracranial atherosclerotic disease. Stenosis of the middle cerebral artery is also a consideration.

4) **What is the prevalence (pretest probability) of each etiology in this patient?**
   The pretest probability of extracranial carotid artery disease in this patient is approximately 15–20%. The prevalence of intracranial stenosis is approximately 5–8%.
5) **What treatment is available for this etiology?**
   For extracranial carotid artery stenosis, carotid endarterectomy is beneficial when the stenosis is greater than 70% by noninvasive imaging or greater than 50% by conventional angiography. For intracranial stenosis, antiplatelet agent is recommended.
6) **What tests/ studies are useful to evaluate this etiology?**
   Given that there is definite treatment evidence for extracranial carotid artery disease and the pretest probability of extracranial carotid disease is high in this patient, evaluating the carotid arteries should be considered first. In a patient where atherosclerosis is thought to be the etiology, as in this patient, carotid ultrasound would provide a high sensitivity and specificity for determining carotid artery stenosis greater than 70%. In addition, it is readily available and relatively inexpensive. If this test did not show significant carotid artery disease, one might consider evaluating the intracranial arteries with MRA or CTA although it might not change management from the default antiplatelet agent and risk-factor management.

CASE 2

A 35-year-old female had been in a minor motor vehicle accident 3 days prior to presentation. Her car was hit from behind and she had a stiff, sore neck. She had been off work the past 3 days. On the day of presentation she developed acute unsteady walking and a novocaine sensation in her right face and her left hand and leg. Her voice became hoarse and she had choked trying to drink water. Her past medical history was significant only for three successful pregnancies and one miscarriage. She was on no medications.

Her examination confirmed the sensory loss of pin prick in the distribution she described. She also had reduced palatal elevation on the right, a smaller pupil on the right as compared to the left with mild right ptosis, and a hemiataxia on the right. Her initial CT scan of the head was negative. Her laboratory studies including CBC, electrolytes, aPTT, PT (INR), and sedimentation rate were normal. Her EKG revealed normal sinus rhythm.

Answering the questions

1) **Is it an ischemic event?**
   The patient's symptoms came on acutely and are in a vascular territory. Therefore one would consider this an ischemic vascular event.

2) **Where does the process localize?**
   This process clearly localizes to the posterior fossa/ posterior circulation and more specifically to the lateral medulla on the right. Remember crossed sensory or motor signs suggest this location, as does a hemiataxia. Horner syndrome can be either in the posterior circulation (affecting the first-order neuron) or anterior circulation (affecting the third-order neuron).

3) **What mechanisms and etiologies are possible?**
   Clues from the history include a recent car accident with neck injury (possible large vessel dissection of the right vertebral artery), patient off work and perhaps sedentary (possible venous clot with paradoxical emboli), and history of miscarriage (possible coagulation disorder).

4) **What is the prevalence (pretest probability) of each etiology in this patient?**

The patient is young and therefore nonatherosclerotic pathologies increase in prevalence. In a young patient, especially with this distribution of infarction, dissection of the vertebral artery is most likely. Some registries suggest that in patients with stroke under 35 years of age, dissection accounts for 10–26% of etiologies. While PFO occurs in one in four people, the onset of symptoms was not with Valsalva and the location of the event is not typical for cardioembolism. Antiphospholipid antibody prevalence in a general population is approximately 2–5%, but accounts for less than 1–4% of ischemic strokes in a general population.

5) **What treatment is available for this etiology?**
   Treatment for dissection is controversial. There are no randomized studies that evaluate whether anticoagulation is better than antiplatelet agents or not, although short-term warfarin is frequently used in clinical practice.

   Paradoxical emboli through a PFO is equally controversial as far as treatment; however if the patient clearly had a lower extremity clot, anticoagulation would be recommended. Coagulation disorders such as Factor V Leiden mutation and prothrombin 20210 mutation generally lead to venous thrombosis and not arterial thrombosis; however, if paradoxical emboli was considered, these may play a role and could affect treatment.

   Anticoagulation is generally used for patients with true antiphospholipid antibody syndrome and ischemic stroke.

6) **What tests/ studies are useful to evaluate this etiology?**
   In this patient, since the pretest probability of dissection is highest and this finding may change management, one would consider beginning with an evaluation of the vertebral arteries with MR or CT angiography of the head and neck. The area of dissection is typically at the high

cervical levels and could be missed with intracranial MRA only. Further studies such as echocardiography or coagulation studies would depend on the result of the initial evaluation.

Conclusion

While there are many tests and procedures available for evaluating and treating cerebrovascular disease, a step-wise evidence-based approach can help to avoid unnecessary risks and costs. Even as diagnostic technologies evolve and new clinical trials are released, the six basic questions will remain helpful when approaching any patient with a potential cerebrovascular ischemic event:

1) Is it a stroke or TIA (versus nonischemic pathology)?
2) Where does the process localize?
3) What mechanisms and etiologies are possible?
4) What is the prevalence (pretest probability) of each etiology in this patient?
5) What treatment is available for this etiology?
6) What tests/ studies are useful to evaluate this etiology?

Selected bibliography

1. Libman R, Wirkowski E, Alvir J, et al. Conditions that mimic stroke in the emergency department. Implications for acute stroke trials. *Arch Neurol* 1995; **52**: 1119–22.
2. Petty G, Brown R, Whisnant JR, et al. Ischemic stroke subtypes: a population-based study of incidence and risk factors. *Stroke* 1999; **30**: 2513–16.
3. Schellinger PD, Bryan RN, Caplan LR, et al. Evidence-based guideline: The role of diffusion and perfusion MRI for the diagnosis of acute ischemic stroke: report of the Therapeutics and Technology Assessment Subcommittee of the American Academy of Neurology. *Neurology* 2010; **75**: 177–85.
4. Furie KL, Kasner SE, Adams RJ, et al. Guidelines for the prevention of stroke in patients with stroke or transient ischemic attack: a guideline for healthcare professionals from the american heart association/ american stroke association. *Stroke* 2011; **42**: 227–76.

5. Ustrell X, Pellise A. Cardiac workup of ischemic stroke. *Curr Cardiol Rev* 2010; **6**: 175–83.
6. Seet RC, Friedman PA, Rabinstein AA. Prolonged rhythm monitoring for the detection of occult paroxysmal atrial fibrillation in ischemic stroke of unknown cause. *Circulation* 2011; **124**: 477–86.
7. Morris J, Duffis E, Fisher M. Cardiac workup of ischemic stroke: can we improve diagnostic yield? *Stroke* 2009; **40**: 2893–8.
8. Harloff A, Handke M, Reinhard M, et al. Therapeutic strategies after examination by transesophageal echocardiography in 503 patients with ischemic stroke. *Stroke* 2006; **37**: 859–64. Erratum in: *Stroke* 2008; **39**: e144.
9. Kapral M, Silver F. Preventive health care, 1999 update: 2. Echocardiography for the detection of a cardiac source of embolus in patients with stroke. Canadian Task Force on Preventive Health Care. *Can Med Assoc J* 1999; **161**: 989–96.
10. Mas J, Arquizan C, Lamy C, et al. Recurrent cerebrovascular events associated with patent foramen ovale, atrial septal aneurysm, or both. *N Engl J Med* 2001; **345**: 1740–6.
11. Huston J, James E, Brown R, et al. Redefined duplex ultrasonographic criteria for diagnosis of carotid artery stenosis. *Mayo Clin Proc* 2000; **75**: 1133–40.
12. Landwehr P, Schulte O, Voshage G. Ultrasound examination of carotid and vertebral arteries. *Eur Radiol* 2001; **11**: 1521–34.
13. Nederkoorn P, Graaf YVD, Hunink M, et al. Duplex ultrasound and magnetic resonance angiography compared with digital subtraction angiography in carotid artery stenosis: a systematic review. *Stroke* 2003; **34**: 1324–32.
14. Kirsch J, Wagner L, James E, et al. Carotid artery occlusion: positive predictive value of duplex sonography compared with arteriography. *J Vasc Surg* 1994; **19**: 642–9.
15. El-Saden S, Grant E, Hathout G, et al. Imaging of the internal carotid artery: the dilemma of total versus near total occlusion. *Radiology* 2001; **221**: 301–8.
16. Brott TG, Halperin JL, Abbara S, et al. Guideline on the management of patients with extracranial carotid and vertebral artery disease: executive summary. *Circulation* 2011; **124**: 489–532.

17. North American Symptomatic Carotid Endarterectomy Trial (NASCET) Investigators. Benefit of carotid endarterectomy for patients with high-grade stenosis of the internal carotid artery. *Stroke* 1991; **22**: 816–17.

18. International Carotid Stenting Study investigators, Ederle J, Dobson J, Featherstone RL, et al. Carotid artery stenting compared with endarterectomy in patients with symptomatic carotid stenosis (International Carotid Stenting Study): an interim analysis of a randomised controlled trial. *Lancet* 2010; **375**: 985–97.

19. Brott TG, Hobson RW 2nd, Howard G, et al., CREST Investigators. Stenting versus endarterectomy for treatment of carotid-artery stenosis. *N Engl J Med* 2010; **363**: 11–23.

20. Powers WJ, Clarke WR, Grubb RL Jr, et al., COSS Investigators. Extracranial-intracranial bypass surgery for stroke prevention in hemodynamic cerebral ischemia: the Carotid Occlusion Surgery Study randomized trial. *JAMA* 2011; **306**: 1983–92.

21. Mohr J, Thompson J, Lazar R, et al. A comparison of warfarin and aspirin for the prevention of recurrent ischemic stroke. *N Engl J Med* 2001; **345**: 1444–51.

22. Roubec M, Kuliha M, Jonszta T, et al. Detection of intracranial arterial stenosis using transcranial color-coded duplex sonography, computed tomographic angiography, and digital subtraction angiography. *J Ultrasound Med* 2011; **30**: 1069–75.

23. Skutta B, Furst G, Eilers J, et al. Intracranial stenoocclusive disease: double detector helical CT angiography versus digital subtraction angiography. *AJNR Am J Neuroradiol* 1999; **20**: 791–9.

24. Chimowitz MI, Lynn MJ, Howlett-Smith H, et al., Warfarin-Aspirin Symptomatic Intracranial Disease Trial Investigators. Comparison of warfarin and aspirin for symptomatic intracranial arterial stenosis. *N Engl J Med* 2005; **352**: 1305–16.

25. Chimowitz MI, Lynn MJ, Derdeyn CP, et al., SAMMPRIS Trial Investigators. Stenting versus aggressive medical therapy for intracranial arterial stenosis. *N Engl J Med* 2011; **365**: 993–1003.

26. Turan TN, Derdeyn CP, Fiorella D, Chimowitz MI. Treatment of atherosclerotic intracranial arterial stenosis. *Stroke* 2009; **40**: 2257–61.

27. Gan R, Sacco R, Kargman DE, et al. Testing the validity of the lacunar hypotehsis: the Northern Manhattan Stroke Study experience. *Neurology* 1997; **48**: 1204–11.

5

Treatment of Hemorrhagic Stroke

Andreas H. Kramer, MD, MSc, FRCPC

Departments of Critical Care Medicine and Clinical Neurosciences, Hotchkiss Brain Institute, Foothills Medical Center, University of Calgary, Alberta, Canada

Intracerebral hemorrhage

Introduction

Intracerebral hemorrhage (ICH) refers to spontaneous bleeding in the brain parenchyma and accounts for about 5–15% of acute strokes. This term should be distinguished from the more general description "intracranial" hemorrhage, which can have numerous subtypes, including bleeding into the subarachnoid, subdural, epidural, and intraventricular spaces.

Epidemiology

The world-wide incidence of ICH is about 20–25 cases per 100,000 person-years. This figure increases dramatically with advancing age and is more common in certain ethnic groups, especially individuals of Asian descent. In the United States, ICH is more common among African-American and Hispanic populations, but this is largely attributable to a higher incidence of hypertension. Another risk factor is lipid levels below population norms.

Etiology

The etiology of ICH can be categorized as being "primary" or "secondary" [1]. Primary ICH refers to spontaneous bleeding that arises because of the fragility of small arterioles in the setting of either chronic hypertension or cerebral amyloid angiopathy (CAA). Secondary ICH refers to hemorrhage that occurs because of anticoagulation or an underlying structural abnormality, such as an arteriovenous malformation (AVM), aneurysm, infarct, or tumor (Table 5.1; Figures 5.1 and 5.2).

Hypertension is by far the most common cause of ICH. The pathological effects of hypertension are most pronounced in the proximal arteriolar branches of penetrating arteries arising from the major vessels at the base of the brain. Thus, hypertensive ICH occurs in characteristic locations, including (in descending order of frequency) the basal ganglia (putamen and caudate nucleus), thalamus, cerebellum, and pons (Figures 5.3, 5.4, and 5.5). The compensatory response that occurs in blood vessels when exposed to persistently high blood pressure (BP) is vascular remodeling with smooth muscle proliferation. Over time, hypertrophied smooth muscle cells develop apoptosis and are replaced by collagen and inflammatory cells. Blood vessels subsequently become ectatic and vulnerable to both hemorrhage (ICH) and occlusion (lacunar infarcts).

CAA is a condition characterized by the deposition of amyloid beta-peptide in the walls of arterioles and capillaries in the cortex and cerebellum. The frequency and severity of CAA increases greatly with age, occurring in almost 10% of individuals older than 75 years. CAA-related ICH is strongly associated with inheritance of certain apolipoprotein E alleles. Hemorrhage attributable to CAA most often occurs in the temporal and occipital lobes. CAA is also thought to be one of the major factors that predispose elderly patients to ICH coincident with anticoagulant use. Patients with either hypertensive or CAA-related ICH often have evidence on gradient echo MRI of satellite microhemorrhages in the corresponding characteristic regions of the brain (Figure 5.6).

Stroke, First Edition. Edited by Kevin M. Barrett and James F. Meschia.
© 2013 John Wiley & Sons, Ltd. Published 2013 by John Wiley & Sons, Ltd.

Table 5.1 Causes of intracerebral hemorrhage and corresponding method of diagnosis

ICH cause	Method of diagnosis
Primary	
Hypertension	Characteristic location, microhemorrhage on GRE MRI
Amyloid angiopathy	Characteristic location, microhemorrhage on GRE MRI
Secondary	
Anticoagulation	Clinical history, atypical location
Arteriovenous malformation	MRI, CT angiogram, catheter angiogram
Cavernous angioma	MRI
Venous angioma	MRI, catheter angiogram
Aneurysm	CT angiogram, catheter angiogram
Neoplasm (primary vs. metastatic)	MRI (with gadolinium)
Venous sinus thrombosis	CT venogram, MR venogram, catheter angiogram
Cocaine, amphetamines	Clinical history, atypical location
Vasculitis	Catheter angiogram, abnormal CSF
Ischemic stroke	CT, DWI MRI

GRE MRI, gradient recall echo magnetic resonance imaging; DWI MRI, diffusion weighted magnetic resonance imaging.

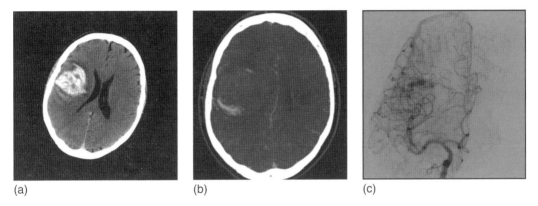

(a)   (b)   (c)

Figure 5.1 Intracerebral hemorrhage (a), complicating an arteriovenous malformation, with corresponding CTA (b) and digital subtraction (c) angiograms.

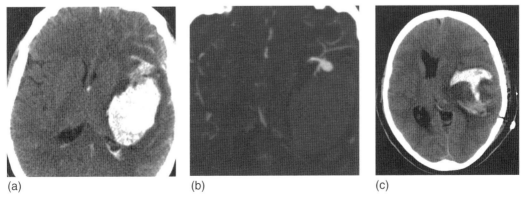

(a)   (b)   (c)

Figure 5.2 Examples of "secondary" intracerebral hemorrhage, including an aneurysm (a, b) and a brain tumor (glioblastoma multiforme) (c).

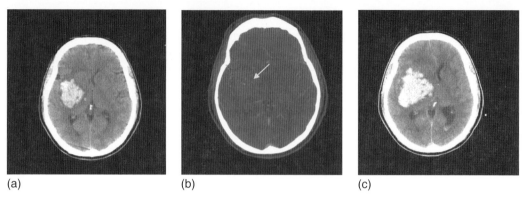

(a)   (b)   (c)

Figure 5.3 Early hematoma expansion complicating ICH. Typical location for hypertensive ICH originating in the putamen (a). The corresponding CT angiogram demonstrates the presence of the "spot sign" (b, arrow). A follow-up CT scan performed 4 hours later reveals substantial hematoma expansion and increasing midline shift (c).

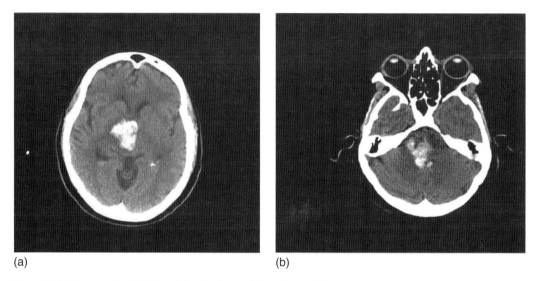

(a)   (b)

Figure 5.4 Hypertensive ICH involving thalamus (a) and pons (b).

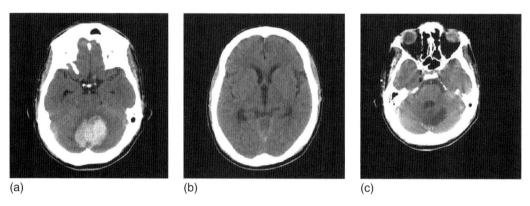

(a)   (b)   (c)

Figure 5.5 Cerebellar ICH complicated by posterior fossa crowding and effacement of the fourth ventricle (a), with resultant obstructive hydrocephalus (b). After evacuation of the hematoma and posterior fossa decompression, the fourth ventricle can again be visualized (c).

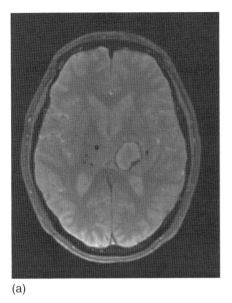 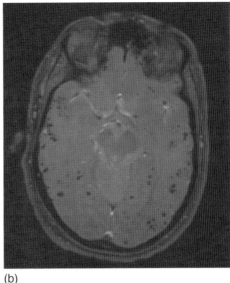

(a)   (b)

Figure 5.6 Gradient echo magnetic resonance imaging (GRE MRI) sequences demonstrating presence of microhemorrhages in a patient with a thalamic hypertensive ICH (a) and cerebral amyloid angiopathy (b). It is common to find microhemorrhages at typical locations remote from the incident hematoma, indicating that chronic vascular disease has preceded the first presentation with ICH.

An increasing proportion of ICH occurs in patients receiving systemic anticoagulation, most often with warfarin. This trend may decline with more widespread use of newer alternative drugs, such as dabigatran and rivaroxaban, which appear to be as efficacious as warfarin in preventing thromboembolic complications, but with a lower rate of ICH. Patients with anticoagulation-induced ICH tend to have larger hematomas and worse outcomes.

Alternative "secondary" causes should be excluded, especially when ICH occurs in young patients or in unusual locations. AVMs are the most common cause of ICH in individuals younger than 40 years. AVMs are a conglomeration of blood vessels in which there is direct communication between the arterial and venous systems, without a normal intervening capillary bed. The veins within AVMs are poorly equipped to withstand the high pressure of the vascular channels that feed into them and are therefore at constant risk of rupture.

Pathophysiology

ICH is a dynamic process whereby hematoma volume increases over a period of hours. Of patients having a CT scan within 3 hours of ICH and a repeat scan after about 24 hours, well over half develop at least some degree of hematoma expansion. The timing of hematoma growth tends to be more protracted in patients receiving anticoagulation. Early hematoma enlargement is strongly associated with worse outcome.

ICH is frequently complicated by surrounding edema, which may progress for as much as 2 weeks following onset of symptoms. Initially, edema forms as serum from the clot moves outwards into the surrounding brain tissue. Subsequently, it may be related to the toxic effects on surrounding brain of hemoglobin and thrombin within the clot. Although cerebral blood flow (CBF) is reduced in the edematous brain tissue around ICH, there generally appears to be a comparable reduction in metabolism, such that classical ischemia is minimal or absent. Reduced metabolism is thought to be attributable to mitochondrial dysfunction. Factors that may contribute to worsening edema include seizures, hyperthermia, and hyperglycemia.

The biochemical mechanisms whereby hemorrhage causes cerebral injury are complex. Apart from the mechanical disruption of neurons and glia, additional pathophysiological factors include the generation of excitatory neurotransmitters such as glutamate, inflammation, disruption of the blood-brain barrier, and apoptosis [2].

Manifestations

The signs and symptoms of ICH are highly dependent on the location of the brain in which it occurs.

Basal ganglia (Figure 5.3)

ICH originating in the putamen usually damages the adjacent internal capsule, thereby causing hemiparesis. Cortical dysfunction may manifest with aphasia (left), hemispatial neglect (right), contralateral hemianopsia, and gaze deviation towards the side of the lesion. The degree to which consciousness is impaired depends especially on the extent of shift of midline structures. Bilateral ptosis is a well-described phenomenon, especially with right hemispheric lesions, and commonly creates the perception that patients are more somnolent than they actually are.

Thalamus (Figure 5.4)

Patients with thalamic ICH are sometimes comatose if the hematoma or surrounding edema extends medially and inferiorly towards the midbrain. In such cases, there may also be corresponding pupillary asymmetry. Consciousness may be regained as edema subsides. Involvement of the midbrain tegmentum or obstructive hydrocephalus from blood in the third ventricle sometimes causes impaired upward gaze. Contralateral hemiparesis is usually present because of damage to the cerebral peduncle or internal capsule. An occasional finding is gaze deviation away from the side of the lesion, a phenomenon referred to as "wrong way eyes." Thalamic hematomas may also produce prominent sensory disturbances. The Dejerine–Roussy syndrome refers to a constellation of features that include pain and sensory loss in the contralateral limbs. A few patients have ICH limited to the anterior regions of the thalamus. These patients are essentially never comatose and usually have a favorable prognosis.

Pons (Figure 5.4)

Pontine ICH frequently has a poor prognosis because of the vital neurological structures and pathways localized to this region. Anterior pontine hemorrhage compromises the corticospinal tracts and leads to various degrees of (quadri-) paresis. Extensor posturing may be observed. Pinpoint pupils occur when there is damage to sympathetic pathways, resulting in bilateral Horner syndrome. A variety of abnormal ocular movements have been described, including "ocular bobbing" (fast downward movement, slow return to primary position), "ocular dipping" (slow downward movement, fast return to primary position), and "ping-pong gaze" (conjugate lateral eye movements from side to side; one cycle every few seconds). Horizontal gaze may be impaired; with unilateral hemorrhage, eyes deviate away from the side of the lesion. Corneal and oculocephalic reflexes are frequently absent. Compression of the cerebral aqueduct may produce obstructive hydrocephalus.

Pontine hemorrhage is usually below the level of the ascending reticular activating system. Thus, although patients are often comatose initially, they may recover consciousness as the rostral edema regresses. It is possible for patients to be awake, but unable to activate facial muscles or move their limbs, a syndrome that is referred to as "locked-in." In its most extreme form, patients can only move their eyes vertically, and it is through this movement that consciousness can be probed.

> **⚠ CAUTION**
>
> Patients who appear comatose with pontine ICH may actually be locked-in. Be sure to ask the patient to look up and down before concluding that they are not conscious. It is sometimes necessary to retract the eyelids to observe volitional vertical eye movements in this context. Inappropriate administration of noxious stimuli may occur if this syndrome is not recognized.

Predictors of poor outcome with pontine ICH include coma at admission, bilateral involvement, relatively larger hematoma volume (diameter >2 cm and volume >4 mL), anterior extension, hydrocephalus, and intraventricular hemorrhage (IVH). Prognosis is generally more favorable when hemorrhage is attributable to a cavernous malformations rather than hypertension.

Cerebellum (Figure 5.5)

Cerebellar ICH is most often attributed to hypertension, but may also occur because of nearby AVMs, aneurysms (posterior inferior cerebellar artery), or brain tumors (usually metastatic). Clinical manifestations commonly include headache, ataxia, nausea, and vomiting. A major concern is the development of edema and mass effect, with resultant life-threatening posterior fossa crowding, brainstem compression, and obstructive hydrocephalus. These complications are more common with hemorrhage into the vermis. While hydrocephalus may contribute to a deteriorating level of consciousness, placement of an external ventricular drain (EVD) is entirely insufficient to alleviate brainstem compression. Instead, surgical decompression is required.

> ### ☝ CAUTION
>
> Cerebellar ICH is a neurosurgical emergency. Patients with cerebellar ICH are at high risk of neurological deterioration. Increasing edema and posterior fossa crowding may cause brainstem compression and obstructive hydrocephalus. Urgent decompressive surgery may be required. Placement of an EVD to treat hydrocephalus is usually insufficient. Patients are at especially high risk if ICH involves the vermis and is >3 cm in diameter.

Although no randomized controlled trials have been published, most investigators have suggested surgical treatment when hematomas have a diameter of more than 3–4 cm, when the quadrigeminal cisterns and/or the fourth ventricle are effaced, or there is a depressed level of consciousness (GCS <13). Emergent evacuation is crucial. Favorable recovery following surgery is less common when patients have already progressed to deep coma with impaired brainstem reflexes.

Intraventricular hemorrhage

IVH occurs in about one-third to one-half of patients, and is strongly associated with more severely impaired consciousness and worse outcomes. The pathophysiological implications of blood in the ventricular system are not well understood, although it appears to induce inflammation and fibrosis, and predispose to the development of acute and chronic hydrocephalus. Hydrocephalus is particularly common when large blood casts occlude the third and fourth ventricles.

Seizures

Convulsive seizures occur in 10 to 20% of patients, most often in the first several hours, and occur more often with cortical ICH. Nonconvulsive seizures may also be common in patients with a persistently impaired level of consciousness, and may contribute to additional neurological injury (Figure 5.7).

Diagnostic considerations

CT scanning remains the most practical, rapid, and readily available modality to diagnose ICH. In the past, angiography was largely reserved for ICH that occurred in young patients (<40 years old) or that had an atypical radiographic location or appearance, suggesting an etiology other than hypertension or CAA. However, CT angiography (CTA) can now easily and efficiently be performed concomitantly with the initial diagnostic noncontrast CT scan. CTAs have reasonable sensitivity and specificity for vascular abnormalities when compared with conventional angiograms. They also enable clinicians to evaluate patients for the presence of a "spot sign," which is emerging as a powerful predictor for subsequent hematoma expansion, and a potential guide for the selection of patients who may benefit from hemostatic therapy (Figure 5.3). The spot sign is present in about a quarter of ICH patients and is associated with larger baseline hematoma volume, a much greater degree of hematoma expansion, and worse neurological outcomes [3]. Routine use of CTAs increases the radiation dose that patients are exposed to, but only rarely results in contrast nephropathy. Catheter angiography still remains a useful test if there is a strong suspicion for a small vascular abnormality despite a normal CT angiogram.

Magnetic resonance imaging (MRI), with use of gradient echo (GRE) sequences, is at least equivalent to CT in the detection of acute ICH (Figures 5.6 and 5.7). MRI can detect cerebral microbleeds, which may help in attributing ICH to hypertension or CAA. MRI may also occasionally allow clinicians to more definitively identify other causes of ICH, such as brain tumors and infarcts [4].

Hematoma volume can be estimated from a CT scan using the ABC/2 system (where A is the greatest hematoma diameter, B is the diameter 90 degrees to A, and C is the approximate number of CT slices with hemorrhage multiplied by the slice thickness). It should be noted that this method is

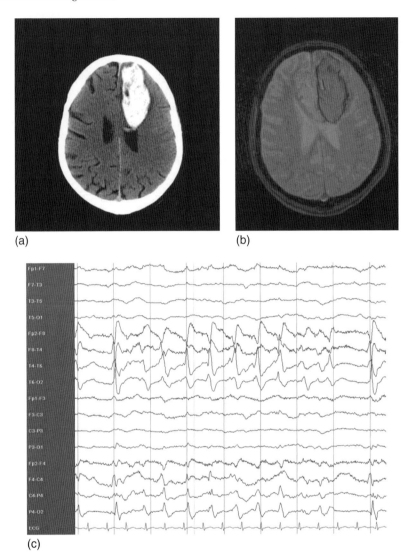

(a)

(b)

(c)

Figure 5.7 CT scan (a) and gradient echo magnetic resonance imaging (GRE MRI) (b) of a patient with left frontal ICH attributable to an arteriovenous malformation. Continuous EEG monitoring (c) demonstrated left hemispheric nonconvulsive status epilepticus.

less accurate when hematomas are not round or ellipsoid, as is often the case with anticoagulation- and thrombolytic-associated ICH.

Treatment

Outcomes following ICH may be improved if patients are cared for in dedicated neurocritical care units. As with other forms of brain injury, care should be directed at limiting any "secondary" damage that may contribute to neurological decline and worse outcomes.

Airway management

Patients with stupor or coma may require endo-tracheal intubation to protect their airway, prevent aspiration, and manage raised intracranial pressure (ICP). As ICH may be in the process of growing at the time of intubation, extreme BP elevation during laryngoscopy should be carefully avoided using an appropriate pharmacological induction strategy (e.g. propofol 1–2 mg/kg), usually with the assistance of neuromuscular blockade (e.g. rocuronium 1 mg/kg). Conversely, until ICP is known, liberal use of sedatives and excessive BP reductions may compromise cerebral perfusion pressure (CPP).

Attenuation of hematoma expansion – hemostatic therapy

Because of the clear relationship between ICH growth and poor outcomes, one would hypothesize that interventions that limit hematoma expansion would improve neurological recovery. However, at present, this hypothesis remains unproven. Since most hematoma growth occurs over only a few hours, the "therapeutic window" for hemostatic therapy is relatively brief, although perhaps somewhat longer in the setting of anticoagulation.

The interaction between tissue factor released at the site of vascular injury and circulating factor VII (FVII) is the crucial initial step in the normal clotting cascade. The potency of exogenously administered recombinant activated FVII (rFVIIa) in promoting thrombin production has generated great interest in its use to limit ICH. Recombinant FVIIa has been evaluated in two large multicenter randomized controlled trials involving patients with spontaneous ICH. When administered at doses of 20–160 µg per kg body weight, rFVIIa did attenuate hematoma growth, but did not improve neurological outcomes [5].

It has been postulated that more selective use of rFVIIa may be required. It may be necessary to restrict it to patients who present earlier and have relatively smaller ICH (where growth can still be prevented). In addition, there are ongoing clinical trials assessing the efficacy of rFVIIa in patients who have a CTA spot sign. Clinicians must be aware that rFVIIa increases the risk of thrombotic complications, especially deep venous thrombosis (DVT).

> ⚝ **TIPS AND TRICKS**
>
> Factor VIIa remains experimental therapy for ICH, even though it has been proven to attenuate hematoma expansion. Patients at highest risk of developing hematoma expansion are most likely to benefit. The CT angiogram "spot sign" identifies such patients. Clinical trials are currently assessing the efficacy of Factor VIIa in this setting. Pending the results of these studies, off-label use could be considered in spot-sign-positive patients who present to hospital early (e.g. <2 hours) and do not have devastatingly large ICH (e.g. >60 mL).

Clotting derangements must be corrected as rapidly as possible in patients with anticoagulation-induced ICH. The most common oral anticoagulant remains warfarin, a vitamin K antagonist. Vitamin K (5–10 mg) should be administered intravenously to all patients. In the past, fresh frozen plasma (FFP) was universally recommended (20–40 mL/kg). Unfortunately, the combination of vitamin K and FFP works relatively slowly. Vitamin K-dependent clotting factors can be replaced more rapidly with a much smaller volume of fluid with the use of prothrombin complex concentrate (PCC). Commercially available PCCs do not require cross-matching or thawing, and can be administered as soon as the INR is noted to be elevated. Rapid INR correction has been demonstrated with four factor (II, VII, IX, and X) preparations; the presence of factor VII may be crucial. The optimal dose of PCC is not known: although 25–50 IU/kg of factor IX activity is usually recommended, as little as 500 IU has been demonstrated to be effective.

> ⚝ **TIPS AND TRICKS**
>
> Appropriate therapy for anticoagulation-induced ICH will be accelerated by rapid detection of the coagulation disturbance. INR testing should be done immediately upon arrival to the emergency department when stroke is suspected. Point-of-care testing devices are increasingly becoming available in emergency departments.

Some clinicians use rFVIIa in the setting of warfarin-induced ICH. Although rFVIIa corrects the INR immediately, it remains unproven that this truly represents normalization of coagulation, rather than simply a laboratory phenomenon. Some animal research suggests that rFVIIa may be less effective than PCC, although reports are conflicting. The most recent American Heart Association (AHA) ICH Guidelines recommend against the use of rFVIIa, and conclude that there is not sufficient evidence at this point to strongly recommend PCC over FFP. Nevertheless, because of the more rapid INR correction with PCC, it is preferred by many clinicians and is now standard in numerous countries.

It is common for patients with ICH to have been receiving antiplatelet drugs, most often aspirin or clopidogrel. Some, but not all, studies have suggested that the degree of hematoma expansion is greater among patients receiving antiplatelet agents. Accordingly, it remains controversial whether hematoma growth can be attenuated by the use of platelet transfusions or platelet-activating drugs (e.g. DDAVP). Our current practice is to administer one dose (4–6 units) of platelets when there is a history of antiplatelet use.

Attenuation of hematoma expansion – blood pressure control

Another potential strategy to limit hematoma expansion is to lower BP during the first several hours after ICH. Acute hypertension is common and is associated with hematoma expansion and worse outcomes. Lingering concerns remain that lowering BP may precipitate ischemia and metabolic distress in the brain tissue surrounding a hematoma. However, this notion has largely not been supported by physiological studies. The multicenter INTERACT trial compared early systolic BP (SBP) goals of 140 versus 180 mmHg and suggested that more aggressive BP control reduced hematoma expansion. This effect was most pronounced among patients with higher baseline BP who were recruited within the first 3 hours after ICH

onset. Ongoing multicenter randomized trials are assessing whether early antihypertensive therapy can improve neurological outcomes [6].

The AHA Guidelines acknowledge that there are incomplete data to guide clinicians. The current recommendation is to consider intravenous antihypertensive infusions when SBP exceeds 200 mmHg or the mean arterial blood pressure (MAP) exceeds 150 mmHg. Modest BP reductions (e.g. SBP ≈ 160/90 mmHg or MAP ≈ 110 mmHg) should be targeted, but clinicians must be cautious if high ICP is suspected, to ensure that CPP remains at least 60 mmHg [7].

If acute hypertension is not responsive to initial pharmacotherapy, or the blood pressure is labile, then an arterial catheter should be placed for continuous monitoring. Short-acting intravenous agents are preferred in order to avoid prolonged, excessive BP reductions beyond the set goal. A number of agents are available and there are no definitive comparative trials suggesting that one drug should be preferred over another (Table 5.2). The most commonly used agents include the beta-blocker labetalol, the calcium-channel blocker nicardipine, and the vasodilators hydralazine and sodium nitroprusside.

Labetalol can be administered as either intermittent doses (10–20 mg every 10–20 minutes) or an

Table 5.2 Intravenous drugs available to treat acute hypertension in hemorrhagic stroke patients

Drug	Dose	Onset	Duration	Precautions
Labetalol	Bolus dosing: 10–40 mg every 10–15 minutes Infusion: 0–2 mg/minute	5–15 minutes	2–4 hours	Accumulates with prolonged infusions Caution using >300 mg total Bradycardia, heart block, LV dysfunction, asthma
Esmolol	0.5–1 mg/kg load then 50–300 µg/kg/min	5 minutes	10–30 minutes	Bradycardia, heart block, LV dysfunction, asthma
Nicardipine	3–15 mg/hour	5–15 minutes	30–60 minutes	Large volume IV fluid at higher rates ICP effects require more study
Nitroprusside	0.25–4 µg/kg/minute	Immediate	1–10 minutes	Cyanide toxicity with prolonged infusions Cerebral vasodilatation and raised ICP
Hydralazine	10–20 mg every 4–6 hours	5–20 minutes	2–6 hours	Reflex tachycardia ICP effects require more study
Enalaprilat	0.625–2.5 mg every 6 hours	15 minutes	4–6 hours	Renal failure, hyperkalemia

LV, left ventricular; ICP, intracranial pressure.

infusion (0–2 mg/minute). Although labetalol is touted as both an alpha- and a beta-blocker, it may still produce life-threatening bradycardia and hypotension if it accumulates. Concern arises especially when the cumulative dose exceeds 300 mg. An alternative, shorter-acting intravenous agent is esmolol. Nicardipine is a dihydropyridine calcium channel blocker that appears safe in the setting of neurological injury, but is currently expensive and must be administered in a relatively large volume of fluid. Sodium nitroprusside is a very effective and short-acting vasodilator. However, many clinicians avoid this drug because of the belief that as a potent cerebral vasodilator it may exacerbate ICP and promote hematoma expansion.

Surgery

Hematoma evacuation with or without suboccipital decompressive craniectomy is indicated for patients with cerebellar ICH and clinical or radiographic evidence of impending brainstem compression (Figure 5.5). In contrast, it is unlikely that surgery is of any benefit among patients with deep brainstem or thalamic ICH. For other supratentorial ICH, the role of surgery is more controversial. Routine surgery was evaluated in the Surgical Trial in Intracerebral Hemorrhage (STICH) [8]. This study compared "early" surgery (median of 20 hours from presentation) with initial conservative treatment. There was no difference in the proportion of patients surviving with a favorable neurological outcome. Importantly, this trial did not specifically evaluate the optimal management of patients with neurological deterioration attributable to increasing edema and midline shift.

One subgroup that may have derived benefit from surgery in the STICH trial was those patients with either cortical ICH or deeper hematomas that projected within 1 cm of the brain surface; this population is currently being evaluated in the STICH II trial. Most other clinical trials of surgery in ICH have been relatively small. None has evaluated surgery beyond 72 hours. A recent Cochrane meta-analysis, based on the results of 10 clinical trials, reported that surgery reduced the odds of death and dependency; however, the results were not robust and differed from the largest published trial (STICH).

A novel surgical approach that is currently being investigated is less invasive, stereotactic hematoma evacuation with the aid of thrombolytics. Such therapy should, however, not be considered standard practice at this time. The AHA Guidelines state that the usefulness of surgery in most cases of ICH is uncertain. At present, standard craniotomy can be considered for patients with moderate-sized lobar clots (>30 mL) within 1 cm of the brain surface.

Intracranial pressure and cerebral physiology

Placement of an ICP monitor is appropriate for most patients with ICH who are comatose. An external ventricular drain (EVD) should be inserted in patients with hydrocephalus, and can also be used as a means of monitoring ICP and treating intracranial hypertension. Other techniques, such as brain tissue oxygen tension ($P_{bt}O_2$) probes or microdialysis catheters, may assist in individualizing treatment targets in selected patients, but have not been well studied with ICH.

Management of raised ICP is similar to the approach used for other types of neurological injury (Table 5.3). Although routine use for all patients is clearly not indicated, both mannitol and hypertonic saline (HTS) have been reported to reduce perihematomal edema and ICP, attenuate metabolic distress, and reverse clinical manifestations of herniation in selected patients.

For patients with IVH, preliminary research demonstrates that use of exogenously administered thrombolytics (e.g. 1 mg tPA every 8–12 hours) can accelerate clearance of blood from the brain. An ongoing multicenter randomized controlled trial is currently assessing the efficacy of this approach at improving neurological outcomes.

Fever

Fever is a common manifestation of ICH, especially in the presence of IVH. Although not studied as extensively as in SAH or ischemic stroke, fever has (inconsistently) been identified as a predictor of worse neurological outcome. Thus, most neurointensivists generally attempt to maintain normothermia. Treatment with acetaminophen (maximum 4 g/day) does lower temperature slightly. If ineffective, a variety of devices are available. For patients who are awake, these strategies may precipitate shivering, which in turn may also have detrimental effects. Apart from antipyretics, a number of other pharmacological agents may have some efficacy in attenuating shivering, including intravenous meperidine, magnesium, dexmedetomidine or

Table 5.3 Prevention and treatment of raised intracranial pressure (ICP)

1. *Most patients*
   Keep head of bed at 30–45 degrees
   If hydrocephalus is present, consider external ventricular drain
   If large ICH, consider surgery in selected cases
   Provide sufficient analgesia: use regular acetaminophen and short-acting opiates; avoid large bolus
       doses
   Ensure that patient is calm: if IV sedatives required, use short-acting drugs (e.g. propofol 0–50 µg/kg/
       minute)
   Ensure that patient is not shivering (see text for therapeutic strategies)
   Rule out nonconvulsive seizures
   Mechanical ventilation targets:
       Po_2 80–120 mmHg
       Pco_2 35–40 mmHg
       Avoid extreme elevations in PEEP (e.g. ≥15 mmHg)
   Other physiological targets:
       Glucose 100–150 mg/dL
       Temperature ≤37.5 °C
       Sodium ≥135 mmol/L
       Hemoglobin ≥8–9 g/dL

2. *If ICP remains elevated*
   Osmotic therapy:
       Mannitol 0.25–1 g/kg every 4-6 hours (ensure osmolar gap normalizes between doses)
       Hypertonic saline (various preparations available; e.g. 2 mL/kg 3–5% saline)
           Monitor [Na⁺] often and keep ≤155 mmol/L
           Carefully avoid rapid reductions in [Na⁺], which may cause "rebound" edema

3. *If ICP still remains elevated (options)*
   Re-consider ICP goals (e.g. ≤25 mmHg rather than ≤20 mmHg may be appropriate)
   Lower Pco_2 (e.g. 28–35 mmHg); consider jugular bulb or $P_{bt}O_2$ monitor to minimize risk of ischemia
   Lower temperature goal (e.g. 35 °C)
   Deeper sedation (e.g. barbiturates or combination of propofol and midazolam); use EEG monitoring
       to guide (e.g. 1–2 bursts per 10 seconds)
   Decompressive surgery

buspirone. One nonpharmacological strategy that may sometimes be effective is the combination of central cooling (e.g. using an endovascular catheter) with surface warming (e.g. using forced-air system); the rationale for this approach is that some afferent temperature receptors are located in the skin of the extremities. There is no proven role for induced hypothermia in ICH. However, preliminary research has suggested that a subphysiological temperature may attenuate perihematomal edema. This strategy could therefore be considered in patients with increasing cerebral edema not responsive to other measures (Table 5.3).

Nosocomial infections

Because nosocomial infections are also prevalent, fever should not be attributed to ICH or IVH until an appropriate work-up has been completed.

Nosocomial pneumonia is a particularly common infection among patients with stroke and impaired consciousness. This probably occurs because of aspiration of gastric contents, but may also be partially attributable to stroke-related impairment of immunity. Some clinicians provide prophylactic antibiotics; however, this approach requires further evaluation before its widespread use can be justified.

Hyperglycemia

Several studies have suggested that hyperglycemia exacerbates the pathophysiology of ICH. Specifically, associations have been demonstrated with hematoma expansion and perihematomal edema. In addition, hyperglycemia may increase the rate of nosocomial infections and has consistently been associated with worse neurological outcomes. On the other hand, glucose metabolism is increased in the zone around a hematoma. Studies utilizing cerebral microdialysis in traumatic brain injury and SAH patients suggest that even moderate reductions in serum glucose may cause pronounced neuroglycopenia. There have been no randomized studies comparing different glucose targets specifically among patients with ICH. However, given that other recent clinical trials have failed to demonstrate any clear benefit from intensive insulin therapy, we currently favor modest glycemic targets (100 to 180 mg/dL).

Seizures

Considering the high prevalence of nonconvulsive seizures reported by some researchers, continuous EEG monitoring may be desirable for ICH patients with stupor or coma. The vast majority of patients who will develop seizures can be identified after 24–48 hours of monitoring. For centers that do not have the resources to do this, repetitive intermittent EEGs are probably preferable to a complete absence of monitoring. There is mounting evidence that non-convulsive seizures are associated with worsened outcomes. Some patients have epileptiform activity without discrete electrographic seizures. The optimal treatment for such EEG patterns, which are part of an "ictal–interictal continuum," is largely unknown. Although seizures are common, recent studies suggest that routine prophylaxis with antiepileptic drugs, especially phenytoin, may not be benign. The AHA Guidelines explicitly recommend against use of prophylactic anticonvulsants. On the other hand, given that seizures may worsen cerebral edema, we do use a short course of prophylactic anticonvulsants in selected patients with significant mass effect.

Anemia

Anemia is relatively common among patients with ICH. As in other critically ill populations, the development of anemia predicts worse outcomes. It remains unproven that such associations are causative and justify the risks associated with more liberal use of red blood cell (RBC) transfusions. The importance of cerebral ischemia as a cause of secondary brain injury in ICH remains controversial. We generally administer RBCs at a hemoglobin concentration of less than 8–9 g/dL in ICH patients, rather than 7 g/dL, which is the usual threshold for most other critically ill patients.

Supportive care – prevention of venous thromboembolism

The incidence of venous thromboembolism in ICH patients has not been well studied, but is probably at least as high as in ischemic stroke patients. Existing studies underestimate the incidence because of a lack of systematic screening. More than with any other condition, concerns about inducing hemorrhagic complications represent a barrier to use of routine pharmacological DVT prophylaxis, at least in the first few days after ICH. Intermittent pneumatic compression stockings (IPCS) should be used in all ICH patients not receiving pharmacological treatment. Some small studies have suggested that it is safe to start subcutaneous low-molecular-weight or unfractionated heparin prophylaxis relatively soon after ICH (e.g. 48 hours). Clearly, the later pharmacological prophylaxis is initiated, the less likely that there will be any consequent hematoma expansion.

Prognostic scales

The most commonly used and best validated prognostic scale is the ICH Score. This system assigns points based on validated prognostic factors, including level of consciousness (Glasgow Coma Scale (GCS) score 3 to 4 = 2 points; GCS score 5 to 12 = 1 point), ICH volume ($\geq 30 \, cm^3$ = 1 point), age (≥ 80 years = 1 point), infratentorial location (1 point), and intraventricular hemorrhage (1 point) [9]. There is a direct relationship between a rising score and mortality. In the study initially describing the ICH score, 30-day mortality rates for patients with scores of 1 to 4 were 13%, 26%, 72%, and 97%, respectively. No patient with a score of 0 died, and none with a score of 5 survived. A score of 6 did not occur, because no patient had the combination of infratentorial location and volume $\geq 30 \, cm^3$. The ICH score has also been validated for longer-term functional outcomes, up to 1 year. Limitations of this score include treating continuous variables (GCS, ICH volume, and age) as categorical, and lumping together of pontine and cerebellar ICH as "infratentorial," even though they may have a quite different prognosis. Recent studies also suggest that the performance of prognostic models may be influenced by the use of "Do Not Resuscitate" (DNR) orders and institutional withdrawal of care practices.

An important consideration in "prognostication" is that patients frequently do continue to improve over the first several months after ICH. That is, the neurological status that is observed in the first few weeks of hospitalization is not perfectly indicative of that patient's potential functional recovery.

End of life care

If the best possible outcome following ICH is to be rendered severely disabled, or perhaps even in a vegetative or minimally conscious state, then many patients would, if given a choice, prefer to forego life-sustaining therapies in an intensive care unit. When such preferences are communicated by surrogate decision makers, the goals of care should generally emphasize comfort and palliation. On the other hand, even with validated prognostic scales like the ICH Score, clinicians' ability to confidently predict long-term neurological prognosis is imperfect. Concern has been expressed by some that clinicians' predictions tend to be excessively pessimistic and that premature withdrawal of life-sustaining interventions may lead to "self-fulfilling prophesies," whereby patients die even though they were not necessarily destined for a dismal outcome. Some have even argued that "early DNR" orders should be avoided altogether [10].

Both of these perspectives are legitimate and need to be carefully balanced. In discussions with patients' surrogate decision makers, it is essential that clinicians be transparent, willing to acknowledge uncertainty, and aware of their influence on decision making. While it is important to avoid unjustified pessimism, patient autonomy must also be respected, and the morbidity and suffering associated with prolonged hospital stays recognized. Different institutions have somewhat varying definitions of what "early DNR" entails and how this impacts on the use of other life-sustaining measures apart from cardiopulmonary resuscitation (CPR). In fact, very few patients with ICH die from unanticipated cardiac arrests. If this does occur in patients who already have severe pre-existing neurological deficits, CPR is, in fact, very unlikely to culminate in a favorable recovery. Introducing limitations in care (e.g. no further surgery, no CPR) is sometimes part of a process whereby patients with a seemingly poor prognosis are still given a "trial of (less aggressive) care."

Subarachnoid hemorrhage

Introduction

Subarachnoid hemorrhage (SAH) is the term used to describe the accumulation of blood between the arachnoid and pia membranes. More than 80% of spontaneous SAH is attributable to ruptured cerebral aneurysms.

Epidemiology

SAH accounts for about 5% of all strokes and has a case fatality rate of 30 to 50%. In North America, the incidence is about 10 cases per 100,000 persons per year, with about two-thirds occurring in women. The prevalence of unruptured intracranial aneurysms in the general adult population is about 3%, but the vast majority of these never become symptomatic.

Etiology

Risk factors for aneurysm formation include a positive family history, smoking, hypertension, and ethanol consumption. The most common locations for aneurysm formation are, in decreasing order, the anterior communicating, internal carotid/ posterior communicating, middle cerebral, basilar, and posterior inferior cerebellar arteries. About a quarter of SAH patients have more than one aneurysm.

The risk that a previously asymptomatic aneurysm will rupture is higher with increasing size, especially when it exceeds 7–10 mm and is located in the posterior circulation. Paradoxically, because small aneurysms are so much more prevalent in the population, and because the relative rate of growth is probably an important factor in the risk of rupture, the majority of patients presenting with SAH have aneurysms smaller than 10 mm.

The most common form of nontraumatic, nonaneurysmal SAH is restricted to the perimesencephalic cisterns, immediately anterior to the brainstem. Perimesencephalic SAH is thought to be venous in origin, and most often has a favorable prognosis. Some cases of SAH where no specific cause is identified may actually be due to ruptured aneurysms that were not visualized on the initial angiogram. False-negative angiograms occur especially when an aneurysm is very small, if it has spontaneously thrombosed, when local vasospasm restricts flow into the aneurysm, or if it is compressed by a surrounding hematoma. In such cases, a repeat angiogram within a week may make the diagnosis. Other rare causes of spontaneous SAH include intracranial arterial dissection, vascular malformations (especially spinal), pituitary apoplexy, and various intracranial vasculopathies (e.g. vasculitis, cerebral vasoconstriction syndromes, or cocaine toxicity) [11].

Pathophysiology

The pathophysiology of SAH is complex and involves both early brain injury (EBI) and later delayed cerebral ischemia (DCI).

Hemorrhage into the subarachnoid space occurs under arterial pressure, resulting in massive, transient elevation of the ICP. The compressing effects of the raised ICP and concomitant, transient acute vasospasm of the ruptured and surrounding vessel(s) usually causes hemorrhage to cease, but may precipitate early ischemic damage. Studies using diffusion-weighted MRI have documented that many patients have infarction even within the first 48 to 72 hours. CBF autoregulation is often impaired, further increasing the vulnerability of the brain to ischemia.

The presence of blood in the subarachnoid space triggers a cascade of biochemical processes. A relative lack of cerebral nitric oxide (NO) is a factor in promoting transient vasoconstriction, platelet aggregation, and inflammation. An excess of the potent vasoconstrictor endothelin-1 is another important contributor to vascular narrowing. Vascular pathology may occur in both large and small vessels, accompanied by damage to the basement membrane, disruption of the blood–brain barrier, and endothelial dysfunction. Cortical spreading depression, where clusters of neuronal depolarization produce an influx of calcium and sodium, results in fluctuations in regional CBF (both hyperemia and ischemia) and brain oxygenation, with possible uncoupling of flow and metabolism. Persistent or recurrent spreading depression may be a major factor associated with both early and delayed cerebral ischemia.

Delayed arterial narrowing, or "vasospasm," occurs in two-thirds of patients, beginning about 72 hours after SAH, and may last for as long as 2 to 3 weeks. The most important risk factors for the development of vasospasm are the amount of blood in the basal cisterns and the initial level of consciousness. The presence of vasospasm is a clear predictor of neurological deterioration, delayed cerebral infarction, and worse outcomes. Some patients with radiographic evidence of severe vasospasm do not become symptomatic. Conversely, some patients deteriorate neurologically despite no more than mild radiographic vasospasm. Thus, the degree to which vasospasm is a direct *cause* of neurological decline, rather than a co-existing process, has been questioned. The pathophysiology of DCI is undoubtedly more complex than being attributable solely to vasospasm, and includes factors such as cortical spreading depression, inflammation, and increased coagulation [12, 13].

Clinical manifestations

The spectrum of clinical manifestations is broad. Some patients present without any neurological deficits; these generally have a favorable prognosis. Others present deeply comatose and may progress to early brain death. About 10 to 15% of patients die prior to reaching hospital.

Almost all conscious patients complain of severe headache, which is usually diffuse, but may be lateralized. The presence of blood and inflammatory cells in the subarachnoid space produces aseptic meningitis, such that patients may have a stiff neck. Nausea and vomiting develop in more than half of cases. A transient loss of consciousness sometimes occurs, coinciding with the transient, massive rise in ICP.

Two grading systems are widely used to describe patients' initial clinical status: the Hunt–Hess and World Federation of Neurological Surgeons (WFNS) scales. Both systems assign scores ranging from 1 to 5; patients with a score of 4 or 5 are commonly referred to as having "high-grade" SAH (Table 5.4). Because it is somewhat more objective and less vulnerable to interobserver variability, we prefer the WFNS system. There is a direct relationship between the clinical grade and eventual outcome.

SAH is a complex, multisystem disorder, which is characterized by the development of a spectrum of life-threatening systemic and neurological complications, which are further described in the section on Treatment.

Diagnostic considerations

With newer-generation CT technology, a noncontrast scan performed within the first 6 to 12 hours has sensitivity for SAH that approaches 100% (Figure 5.8). This sensitivity decreases substantially

Table 5.4 Clinical scales used to grade patients with subarachnoid hemorrhage

	Hunt–Hess	WFNS
I	Asymptomatic or mild headache	GCS score 15 without hemiparesis
II	Moderate to severe headache, nuchal rigidity, no focal deficits other than cranial nerve palsy	GCS score 13–14 without hemiparesis
III	Confusion, lethargy, or mild focal deficits other than cranial nerve palsy	GCS score 13–14 with hemiparesis
IV	Stupor or moderate to severe hemiparesis	GCS score 7–12
V	Coma, extensor posturing, moribund appearance	GCS score 3–6

GCS, Glasgow Coma Scale; WFNS, World Federation of Neurological Surgeons score.

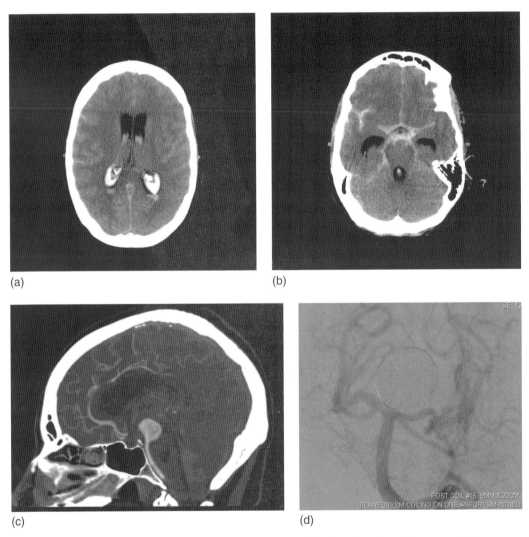

(a)

(b)

(c)

(d)

Figure 5.8 CT scans and catheter angiograms of a patient with subarachnoid and intraventricular hemorrhage (a,b) due to a large, ruptured basilar artery tip aneurysm (c,d). There is also ventriculomegaly consistent with hydrocephalus. The aneurysm was managed with endovascular coil embolization (d).

over the subsequent week. Thus, if patients present to hospital several days after onset of a headache, and clinical suspicion remains high despite a "negative" CT scan, a lumbar puncture should be performed to look for red blood cells and xanthochromia, the discoloration of CSF that occurs because of hemoglobin degradation products. Xanthochromia develops after about 2 to 4 hours and can be detected for as long as 2 weeks after SAH. The most common reason for a diagnosis of SAH to be missed is that a CT scan is not performed, most often because patients present with a normal level of consciousness and their headache is wrongly attributed to other causes.

✋ CAUTION

CT scans are very sensitive for SAH, but only if they are performed within the first 1 to 2 days. If patients present with a more prolonged history of headache and a normal CT scan, a lumbar puncture should be considered.

The quantity of subarachnoid and intraventricular blood visible on the initial CT scan is a major predictor for the development of subsequent complications, especially DCI. Historically, the most common system used to quantify the relative amount of blood has been the Fisher scale. This scale was developed at a time when on-line computerized images were not yet available, and the dimensions on X-ray films were smaller than actual size. Subarachnoid clots were interpreted as "thick" if the width exceeded 1 mm. In reality, it is uncommon for clots to be less than 1 mm thick. It is also unclear from the original description whether patients with "thick" SAH and IVH should be given a Fisher score of 3 or 4. To overcome these limitations, a modified version has been proposed and validated as being more predictive of complications than the original Fisher score (Table 5.5).

Once SAH has been diagnosed, the next step is to identify the source of bleeding (Figure 5.8). Although catheter angiography remains the gold standard for diagnosis of cerebral aneurysms, CTA has comparable sensitivity and is sufficient in the majority of cases, especially when aneurysms exceed 4 mm in diameter. Recent CT technology also enables three-dimensional re-construction of

Table 5.5 Radiographic scales used to grade patients with subarachnoid hemorrhage

	Fisher Scale	Modified Fisher Scale
0		No SAH or IVH
1	No SAH or IVH	Minimum* or thin SAH, no IVH
2	Diffuse, thin SAH, no clot >1 mm in thickness	Minimum or thin SAH, with IVH
3	Localized thick subarachnoid clot >1 mm in thickness	Thick SAH, no IVH
4	Predominant IVH or intracerebral hemorrhage without thick SAH	Thick SAH, with IVH

* The definition of "thick" is at least 5 mm.
IVH, intraventricular hemorrhage; SAH, subarachnoid hemorrhage.

aneurysms for surgical planning. If the CTA does not reveal an aneurysm, then a catheter angiogram should still be arranged. If this is also negative, a repeat study after approximately 1 week should be performed. If subarachnoid blood is seen primarily in the posterior fossa, then an MRI should be considered to exclude a spinal vascular malformation or aneurysm.

Treatment

As in other critically ill populations, outcomes of patients with SAH appear to be better at experienced, high-volume centers. It is likely that the multidisciplinary expertise provided at such centers, as well as the use of an organized, consistent approach, is largely responsible for superior outcomes. Consensus guidelines for the critical care management of patients with SAH have recently been published by the Neurocritical Care Society. Treatment priorities tend to differ somewhat in the earlier (initial 48–72 hours) versus later phases [14, 15].

Initial 48–72 hours – cardiopulmonary support

It is common for patients with high-grade SAH to exhibit significant cardiopulmonary instability during the initial several hours. Meticulous critical care is required during this crucial phase to minimize secondary brain injury and maximize the chance of a favorable neurological recovery.

Airway management

For patients requiring endotracheal intubation, clinicians must balance concerns about aneurysm rebleeding, raised ICP, cerebral ischemia, and cardiac dysfunction. Thus, the aim during intubation should be to minimize fluctuations in BP and to avoid increments in ICP. Blood pressure should be monitored carefully, ideally with an arterial catheter. Vasoactive drugs (e.g. phenylephrine) should be available in case BP drops more than intended.

Neurogenic pulmonary edema

A substantial proportion of patients with high-grade SAH present with bilateral pulmonary infiltrates and impaired gas exchange. In some cases, this may be attributable to aspiration pneumonitis. More commonly, it is due to neurogenic pulmonary edema. This condition is thought to arise because of a combination of increased pulmonary capillary hydrostatic pressure and permeability. High pressures occur because of concomitant cardiac dysfunction and sympathetically mediated acute pulmonary venoconstriction. The mechanism responsible for increased permeability is less certain, but may be partially attributable to damage induced by the rapid rise in pulmonary capillary pressure that occurs at the time of SAH (the "blast theory").

Patients with neurogenic pulmonary edema may develop profound hypoxemic respiratory failure. Although the initial presentation is similar to that of acute lung injury (ALI) or acute respiratory distress syndrome (ARDS), the natural history usually differs, with improvements occurring relatively quickly over the first few days. Treatment is supportive, as there is no proven pharmacological therapy. Unlike the usual ventilatory management of ALI/ARDS, clinicians should be careful to avoid not only hypoxemia, but also hypercapnia, which produces cerebral vasodilatation and elevations in ICP.

Neurogenic stunned myocardium

A variety of electrocardiographic abnormalities may occur after SAH, including QT prolongation and ST segment and T wave changes. Elevation of cardiac troponin levels occurs in approximately 20% of patients overall; importantly, this includes 30–40% of Hunt–Hess grade 4 patients and 75–80% of grade 5 patients. In most such cases, there will also be significant elevations in plasma B-type natriuretic peptide levels and echocardiographic evidence of left ventricular dysfunction. The mechanism is thought to involve massive catecholamine release from myocardial sympathetic nerve endings, which in turn induces myocardial band necrosis. Although some patients present with a pattern consistent with takotsubo syndrome (with prominent apical hypokinesis), it is more common to have relative apical sparing, consistent with the sympathetic innervation within the heart. Wall motion abnormalities generally do not follow typical coronary artery disease distributions. If patients can be successfully supported, the prognosis from neurogenic stunned myocardium is generally favorable, with relatively rapid improvement in cardiac function over the ensuing week.

Initial hemodynamic goals must balance competing interests. On the one hand, a lower BP will help optimize cardiac performance. Conversely, ICP may be elevated, such that conventional BP goals are insufficient to maintain adequate CPP. We generally target the lowest BP goal possible that will still ensure a CPP of at least 60 to 70 mmHg. CPP is the difference between mean arterial blood pressure and ICP. For patients who are hypotensive because of neurogenic stunned myocardium, it seems prudent to avoid supporting them with the pure alpha agonist phenylephrine, which raises afterload, and instead use an agent with at least some beta-receptor stimulation. Given that norepinephrine raises CBF more predictably than dopamine, it is our preferred vasopressor (0.01–0.50 μg/kg/minute). However, we combine this with dobutamine or milrinone, as necessary, to augment cardiac output.

Initial 48–72 hours – neurological resuscitation
Hydrocephalus
The prevalence of acute hydrocephalus following SAH is about 20 to 30%. Hydrocephalus develops because blood, inflammatory cells, and adhesions block CSF absorption at the arachnoid granulations. Accordingly, radiographic and clinical evidence of hydrocephalus is especially common among patients with a poor clinical grade and relatively large amounts of subarachnoid and intraventricular blood.

A sizable proportion of poor-grade SAH patients will show neurological improvement after placement of an external ventricular drain (EVD). Some patients will improve even if the degree of ventriculomegaly observed radiographically is not impressive; thus, it is our practice to place an EVD in essentially all patients with coma. In selected cases, when there is communicating hydrocephalus, use of a lumbar drain or large volume lumbar puncture may be a reasonable alternative. Patients may have ventriculomegaly and a depressed level of consciousness even if the ICP is not especially high.

Concern has been expressed that CSF drainage could theoretically create a trans-aneurysmal pressure gradient, which could in turn increase the risk of rebleeding if performed prior to definitive treatment. More recent studies have not supported this concept and we do not believe that this theoretical concern should prevent clinicians from placing an EVD. However, when an EVD is inserted, "excessive" drainage of CSF should probably be avoided. Thus, the level of the EVD should initially be set no lower than 10 to 15 cm H_2O above the external auditory meatus. While some authors prefer that EVDs be placed in the operating room to reduce the risk of infection, most literature has reported that the rate of catheter-related infections is comparable when they are placed in the intensive care unit.

Cerebral edema and raised intracranial pressure
EVD placement enables clinicians to monitor ICP and, unlike other forms of pressure monitoring, provides a means of lowering ICP through controlled drainage. Patients with high-grade SAH commonly develop global cerebral edema. Focal ICH and surrounding edema may cause regional mass effect, brain tissue shifts, and high ICP. Raised ICP (>20 mmHg) is associated with worse outcomes, especially if it is not responsive to therapy. Treatment of raised ICP is described in Table 5.3.

Prevention of rebleeding
Recurrent hemorrhage from a previously ruptured aneurysm is one of the most devastating complications following SAH. The prevalence of rebleeding is reported to be about 5 to 25%. This figure has been underestimated in the literature, since ultra-early rebleeding occurring within the first several hours may easily be missed. The mortality rate associated with rebleeding is greater than 50%. The highest risk is in the first several hours after the ictus, before most centers can realistically treat an aneurysm.

Antifibrinolytic drugs
In the era preceding routine aneurysm surgery, it was common practice to administer antifibrinolytic agents for 1 to 2 weeks to minimize the risk of rebleeding. This practice was clearly demonstrated in randomized controlled trials to be efficacious in reducing rebleeding. Unfortunately, antifibrinolytic agents also appeared to increase the rate of DCI and infarction, thereby offsetting any potential benefit. However, there have been major changes in practice since most of these studies were performed. First, aneurysms are now routinely secured within the initial 48 hours post SAH; thus, the required duration of antifibrinolytic therapy is much shorter and does not extend into the period of maximal DCI risk. Second, nimodipine is now routinely administered as a neuroprotective agent. Finally, it is no longer common to utilize volume depletion as a means of preventing rebleeding or lowering ICP; this practice has been linked with a higher risk of DCI. More recent randomized controlled trials have suggested that antifibrinolytics reduce rebleeding rates without increasing concerns about DCI. Although clinical trials have not definitively proven that antifibrinolytics improve neurological outcomes, we believe that use of antifibrinolytic agents should be considered in selected patients at particularly high risk of rebleeding in whom surgical or endovascular therapy will be delayed by more than 6 to 12 hours. The optimal drug to use remains unclear, although tranexamic acid is more potent than epsilon aminocaproic acid and was utilized in the most promising clinical trial, where it was administered at an initial intravenous dose of 1 gram, which can be repeated every 6 to 8 hours until the aneurysm has been definitively treated.

★ TIPS AND TRICKS
If definitive aneurysm treatment (clipping or coiling) will be delayed more than a few hours, consider administering 1 gram of tranexamic acid to reduce the risk of rebleeding.

Blood pressure control

High blood pressure is very common in the first several hours after SAH. Some studies have suggested that a higher BP is associated with a greater risk of rebleeding. However, there are no randomized studies indicating that this risk can be offset by aggressive BP treatment. While there is a strong theoretical rationale, excessive BP reductions may precipitate cerebral ischemia. Particular caution is required when the ICP is not known, but likely to be elevated.

Consistent with the Neurocritical Care Society Guidelines, we generally aim to keep the SBP below 160 mmHg and MAP below 110 mmHg. We also strive to keep the CPP above 60 mmHg in most patients, and above 70 mmHg in those with chronic hypertension. These goals only apply until the aneurysm has been secured, after which BP should no longer be lowered deliberately.

In combination, the provision of adequate analgesia, treatment of anxiety, and initiation of nimodipine (see below) are often sufficient to control BP without the need for any additional pharmacological agents. If further therapy is required, the optimal drug choice is uncertain (Table 5.2). As with ICH, we generally avoid nitroprusside. For patients with preserved cardiac function and without bradycardia, labetalol and esmolol are reasonable options. Nicardipine is another safe alternative; the main barrier to its more widespread use is cost.

Definitive aneurysm treatment

The two methods of treating cerebral aneurysms are surgical clip ligation and endovascular coil embolization. The endovascular approach is clearly preferred for treatment of posterior circulation aneurysms, especially those involving the basilar artery (Figure 5.8). An increasing proportion of other patients are also being managed with an endovascular approach. This paradigm shift was supported by the ISAT trial, a randomized comparison that reported a 7% absolute risk reduction in mortality (number needed to treat 15) among patients treated endovascularly in whom there was equipoise concerning the most appropriate intervention.

Clipping and coiling should be regarded as complimentary methods. In patients with significant ICH, as may occur especially with anterior communicating and middle cerebral artery aneurysms, a craniotomy allows both evacuation of clot and definitive treatment of the aneurysm. The morphology of certain aneurysms may also make one method more suitable than another. Large-volume centers must have expertise in both modes of therapy and treatment decisions are increasingly made by consensus.

Perioperative considerations

Prior to final placement of a surgical clip, vascular neurosurgeons must often temporarily occlude the parent artery, sometimes repeatedly. Also, it is not uncommon for flow through small perforator vessels arising from the corresponding vessel to be compromised by placement of the final clip. For these reasons, early infarction is a potential postoperative complication. Risk factors for infarction include the maximum and total duration of temporary vessel occlusion, as well as the number of clips applied. Particularly with middle cerebral artery (MCA) or internal carotid artery aneurysms, infarction may, in turn, result in worsening mass effect and midline shift. Concerns about these complications should prompt early postoperative imaging.

Lumbar drainage is sometimes performed during aneurysm surgery to facilitate brain relaxation for improved surgical exposure. In some patients, this may predispose to the development of CSF hypovolemia with consequent "brain sag," characterized by neurological deterioration and features of transtentorial herniation. CT scans typically reveal effacement of the basal cisterns and an oblong appearance of the brainstem. Recognition of this syndrome is important, because the usual therapies used to treat intracranial hypertension may be ineffective. Patients should generally be placed into the Trendelenburg position. Consultation with the anesthesia service for performance of an epidural blood patch, to prevent ongoing CSF leakage, can be considered.

The most feared complication during endovascular therapy is aneurysm rupture during placement of the coils. Anticoagulants, such as intravenous heparin, and antiplatelet drugs, such as abciximab, are sometimes administered during coiling. Intensivists must be aware of the lingering presence of these drugs in the immediate postoperative period, to ensure that other invasive procedures are appropriately delayed.

Beyond 72 hours

Prevention of delayed cerebral ischemia

Clinicians should avoid using the terms vasospasm and DCI interchangeably. Vasospasm is a radiographic diagnosis, which most often does not require specific therapy other than vigilance in rapidly detecting cerebral ischemia if it occurs. DCI refers to delayed neurological deterioration, which may in some cases be directly attributable to vasospasm, but may also have other pathophysiological contributors.

Patients with SAH commonly "waste" sodium in urine and are therefore prone to becoming volume depleted. Hypovolemia may predispose patients to the development of DCI, and should therefore be carefully avoided. Conversely, aggressive volume expansion, targeting supranormal central venous pressure, has little impact on CBF or DCI, may reduce $P_{bt}O_2$ and increases complications.

Nimodipine is a calcium channel blocker that reduces the risk of DCI and improves outcomes after SAH. The mechanism of neuroprotection may not be related to amelioration of vasospasm. The usual dose is 60 mg, administered enterally every 4 hours. In patients where nimodipine lowers blood pressure excessively, the dosing regimen can be modified to 30 mg every 2 hours. The duration of therapy has ranged from 14 to 21 days in clinical trials.

Statins are a drug class with pleiotropic effects, several of which could help prevent DCI. Several small, single-center randomized controlled trials seem to suggest that statins reduce DCI. However, the results of trials have been inconsistent, and observational data, involving a much larger number of patients, does not confirm the effectiveness of statins. In addition, statins have not yet convincingly been shown to have any impact on neurological outcomes. Thus, while individual centers may choose to use them, statins should not be regarded as standard care.

The central importance of endothelin 1 in the pathogenesis of cerebral vasospasm was the rationale for recent clinical trials involving endothelin-receptor antagonists (ETRAs) in the prevention of DCI. Although very effective at ameliorating vasospasm, ETRAs do not appear to improve neurological outcomes. It is possible that adverse effects of these drugs may offset some of the benefit. Alternatively, DCI occurs by mechanisms other than only vasospasm, and these pathways may not be sufficiently modified.

Magnesium has been proposed as a therapy to prevent DCI. It has numerous potential neuroprotective mechanisms, including vasodilatation, reduced glutamate toxicity, and calcium channel blockade. While some studies has suggests a reduction in DCI, there is no proven effect on neurological outcomes. Our practice is to be vigilant in avoiding hypomagnesemia, but we do not use additional magnesium supplementation.

Diagnosis of delayed cerebral ischemia

The most basic approach to monitoring is simply repeated neurological assessments. DCI may produce both focal deficits and alterations of consciousness. This is more challenging to detect in higher-grade patients, where neurological deterioration may be more subtle. Clinicians must be aware that some patients develop cerebral infarction without first developing easily detectable neurological manifestations.

Most ancillary monitoring is aimed at the diagnosis of large vessel vasospasm. It is unclear how common it is for patients to develop true DCI without *any* vasospasm. In the CONSCIOUS study, where all patients underwent catheter angiography on day 8 ± 2, this was relatively rare, although the severity of vascular narrowing in patients with confirmed DCI was sometimes only mild.

A relatively large number of studies have compared transcranial Doppler (TCD) with catheter angiography for the detection of vasospasm. Cumulatively, these studies suggest that TCD is more specific than it is sensitive. There are much more data concerning the diagnostic accuracy of TCD for detection of MCA vasospasm compared with other vessels. The sensitivity and specificity for MCA vasospasm have been reported to be 38 to 91% and 94 to 100%, respectively. Values for other vessels are less certain. We find daily TCD monitoring especially useful among patients in whom the baseline neurological examination is abnormal.

Mild TCD vasospasm is generally defined by a MCA mean flow velocity of 120 to 160 cm per second. The criteria for moderate and severe vasospasm are 160 to 200 cm/second and >200 cm/second, respectively. However, MCA velocities should always be interpreted in combination with ICA velocities. The ratio of MCA/ICA velocity is referred to as the Lindegaard Ratio. With vasospasm, this ratio is generally elevated (mild if >3, severe if

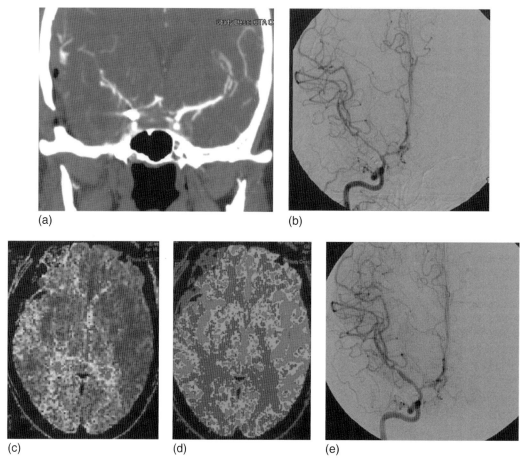

(a)   (b)

(c)   (d)   (e)

Figure 5.9 CT and catheter angiogram images (a,b) demonstrating right middle cerebral artery (MCA) vasospasm 6 days after a ruptured right posterior communicating artery aneurysm. The CT perfusion images (c,d) show increased mean transit time (c) and reduced blood flow (d) in the right MCA vascular territory. Vasospasm was treated with balloon angioplasty (e). (See also Plate 5.9).

>6). If both values are elevated, but the ratio is unchanged, this is more consistent with hyperemia.

The gold standard for detection of vasospasm is catheter angiography. This is an invasive modality that is not always available in a timely fashion, especially overnight or on weekends. In contrast, CT angiography is noninvasive, readily available, and has excellent sensitivity and specificity for vasospasm (Figure 5.9). The accuracy of magnetic resonance angiography is less well established.

Angiography does not provide information concerning the physiological implications of arterial narrowing. This may make the findings of vascular imaging difficult to interpret. Some patients with severe vasospasm remain asymptomatic, such that aggressive interventions (which have potential complications) may not be justified. Alternatively, some patients with only moderate vasospasm may develop cerebral ischemia necessitating more aggressive therapy. Thus, imaging modalities that provide information concerning cerebral perfusion may provide important complimentary information to vascular imaging. CT perfusion (CTP) studies can easily be performed immediately following CTAs, without the need for additional patient transport (Figure 5.9).

Preliminary research suggests that CTP has a greater sensitivity and specificity for DCI than CTA or catheter angiography alone. Abnormalities detected using CTP in patients with DCI appear to be reversible with therapy in many patients.

★ TIPS AND TRICKS

Consider obtaining a CT perfusion scan to complement information derived from CT angiography. This may be especially helpful in clarifying the physiological relevance of mild–moderate vasospasm and determining whether aggressive therapy is justified.

Additional investigational methods that have been proposed to detect DCI include $P_{bt}O_2$, microdialysis, and quantitative cEEG monitoring, but further research is required before these can be considered standard.

Treatment of delayed cerebral ischemia

Several case series have described the use of so-called "triple H" therapy, referring to "hypervolemia," "hemodilution," and "hypertension," with clinical improvement reported in about two-thirds of patients. While hypovolemia should be strictly avoided, recent studies suggest that supra-normal volume expansion has little benefit. Although hemodilution does increase CBF, the reduction in arterial oxygen content induced by a lower Hb results in an overall decrement in cerebral oxygen delivery. In contrast, induced hypertension has convincingly been demonstrated to raise CBF and improve cerebral oxygenation, and in some cases to improve neurological status. Increments in CBF may occur especially in regions of the brain that are affected by arterial vasospasm. Thus, the initial therapeutic approach targets normovolemia, an "adequate" Hb concentration, and a higher blood pressure. We prefer the terms "hemodynamic augmentation" or "induced hypertension" rather than "triple H therapy."

There are no randomized trials that have investigated the use of hemodynamic augmentation as treatment for patients diagnosed with DCI. The only (negative) trials assessing the utility of such therapy have been performed in a prophylactic fashion prior to the development of DCI. Given that induced hypertension has potentially deleterious effects, we favor a step-wise strategy, whereby BP is raised in gradual increments, with frequent re-evaluation of the therapeutic goals. For example, an initial approach might be to raise the MAP by 10 to 15% and then repeat a neurological assessment to determine if there has been any improvement.

The implications of induced hypertension on cardiac performance should also be carefully monitored. Optimal BP goals will likely vary from one patient to another. We are particularly careful in using hemodynamic augmentation in patients with only mild–moderate radiographic vasospasm, without other convincing evidence for cerebral ischemia. CTP studies may be useful in making this judgment. If induced hypertension has no effect on a patient's clinical status, or cerebral vasospasm is in the process of resolving, then gradual "weaning" of therapy should be considered. Another method of increasing CBF in the context of vasospasm is to raise cardiac output with inotropes. Both dobutamine and milrinone have been used for this purpose.

If patients do not improve with hemodynamic augmentation, and there is moderate–severe vasospasm in vascular territories that could explain the deterioration, then endovascular therapy can be attempted. With focal, proximal narrowing, angioplasty is preferred, since it has a relatively durable effect (Figure 5.9). Alternatively, several drugs can be administered intra-arterially to improve vascular caliber. Agents that have been used for this purpose include papaverine, nicardipine, verapamil, and milrinone. There have been no randomized controlled trials of these interventions. In each case, the impact of intra-arterial therapy is relatively transient, such that the procedure may need to be repeated.

Seizure prophylaxis and treatment

Seizures are not uncommon following SAH, most often shortly after the onset. Patients also frequently experience spontaneous posturing, which may be misinterpreted as a seizure. Subsequent seizures during hospitalization are less common, occurring in 2 to 7% of patients. Risk factors that have been identified include: worse neurological grade, larger cisternal clot burden, the presence of ICH, MCA aneurysm location, hydrocephalus, and DCI.

When aggressively sought using cEEG monitoring, nonconvulsive status epilepticus may be relatively common, occurring in as many as 10% of patients. This possibility should be considered in any patient with unexplained neurological deterioration.

Because phenytoin has been associated with worse neurocognitive recovery in SAH patients, we do not use it routinely for seizure prophylaxis. Whether there is any clinical benefit to using alternative prophylactic anticonvulsant drugs requires further study. Some clinicians administer anticonvulsants prophylactically for 48 to 72 hours, until the aneurysm has been secured.

Fever

Fever occurs in more than half of patients with SAH. The average daily maximum temperature is more than 1 °C above normal (37 °C). The strongest predictors of fever include higher neurological grade, larger amounts of intracranial blood, and the presence of IVH. Numerous studies have reported an association between fever and both delayed infarction and worse outcomes.

Treatment of fever was discussed in the section on ICH. In animal studies, hyperthermia is extremely deleterious in the setting of cerebral ischemia. Because one of the major goals in caring for patients with SAH is to prevent DCI, temperature control is particularly important in this setting.

Anemia

The circulating concentration of hemoglobin is a major determinant of oxygen delivery to the brain. A large body of literature has demonstrated an association between anemia and worse outcomes in SAH patients. Studies utilizing multimodal monitoring have shown that lower hemoglobin concentrations are associated with critically low $P_{bt}O_2$ values and metabolic distress. A study using PET scanning has reported that RBC transfusion may increase oxygen delivery and improve the ischemic tolerance in oligemic regions of the brain.

Many clinicians are more liberal in their use of RBCs among high-grade SAH patients and those with vasospasm, especially when it is symptomatic. Our practice is to transfuse when hemoglobin concentrations fall below 9 to 10 g/dL in patients with vasospasm or DCI. In asymptomatic patients, we consider a threshold hemoglobin concentration of 7 to 8 g/dL to be appropriate.

Hyperglycemia

Observational studies suggest that hyperglycemia is associated with worse outcomes in SAH patients. The mechanism for such an association remains uncertain. A small clinical trial performed in SAH patients reported that intensive glycemic control (goal 80 to 110 mg/dL) rather than "loose" control (goal <220 mg/dL) reduced nosocomial infections, but had no effect on neurological recovery. As with ICH, we target glucose concentrations of 100 to 180 mg/dL and are vigilant in avoiding hypoglycemia.

Hyponatremia

Hyponatremia is the most common electrolyte disturbance following SAH, occurring in about one-third of patients. It is thought to be primarily attributable to the cerebral salt wasting syndrome, which is caused by high levels of natriuretic peptides. The "syndrome of inappropriate antidiuretic hormone secretion" (SIADH) may also play a role. These two entities are difficult to distinguish. Although mild hyponatremia (e.g. 125 to 135 mmol/L) does not necessarily require treatment in other critically ill populations, it is not well tolerated in the context of SAH. SAH patients frequently have cerebral edema, which may be exacerbated by hyponatremia, and the consequent reduction in osmolarity. Hyponatremia may increase the risk of seizures in patients who already have a particular vulnerability. Subtle alterations in neurological status attributable to hyponatremia could be misinterpreted as being due to DCI or other causes, thereby potentially precipitating unnecessary investigations and treatments.

Sodium levels should be measured at least once daily. Hypotonic solutions (e.g. 0.45% saline) should be strictly avoided and intravenous medications should be prepared in normal saline rather than hypotonic dextrose solutions. In patients who develop hyponatremia despite maintenance of adequate circulatory volume, our next step is use of hypertonic saline (1.8 to 3%), initially at a rate of 25 to 50 mL/hour, with the goal of keeping the sodium concentration at least 135 mmol/L. In patients with high ICP, a higher goal (e.g. >140 to 145 mmol/L) could be considered. Central venous access is preferred because of the potential for hypertonic saline to cause phlebitis. Fluid restriction is dangerous, and should not be used, even if clinicians believe the etiology to be SIADH. Potential complications of hypertonic saline include volume overload, hypokalemia from renal potassium wasting, and the development of hyperchloremic metabolic acidosis. Rapid reversal of hyponatremia may predispose patients to the development of osmotic demyelination. For all patients receiving hypertonic saline, serum electrolytes should be assessed on a regular basis (e.g. every 4 to 8 hours). If iatrogenic *hyper*natremia has been present for more than 12 to 24 hours, then rapid reductions (>0.3 mmol/L/hour) should be carefully avoided, especially in patients with cerebral edema.

In situations where clinicians want to avoid hypertonic saline (e.g. concerns about cardiac dysfunction, fluid overload, or lack of central venous access), the mineralocorticoid fludrocortisone has been shown to attenuate sodium wasting and hyponatremia. Use of the intravenous vasopressin receptor antagonist conivaptan is increasingly being reported in neurocritical care patients, but its specific role remains to be defined.

DVT prophylaxis

Some literature has reported DVTs to be very prevalent in SAH, especially among high-grade patients. Mechanical prophylaxis should be used in all patients on admission. Because of the dire implications of rebleeding, most clinicians would not initiate pharmacological prophylaxis until clipping or coiling has been performed. Even after aneurysm treatment, clinicians must be aware that patients may undergo other invasive procedures, including lumbar punctures and EVD placement or removal. For this reason, and because of concerning trends towards more intracranial hemorrhagic complications observed in small clinical trials with low-molecular-weight heparin, we currently favor unfractionated heparin in most SAH patients.

Prognosis

Increasing age, higher neurological grade, larger amounts of blood on CT scans, and the presence of intracerebral or intraventricular hemorrhage are all factors that have been consistently demonstrated to be associated with worse outcomes in multivariable models. None of these, on their own, are sufficiently definitive to justify early withdrawal of life-sustaining therapies. Among patients with WFNS or Hunt–Hess grade V SAH who are deeply comatose, neurosurgeons may initially defer aneurysm treatment, and proceed only if patients demonstrate some improvement over the ensuing 48 to 72 hours. Despite the high risk of rebleeding, the rationale for this approach is that outcomes in cohort studies have generally been dismal for patients whose motor response does not improve beyond a motor score of 3 (flexor posturing) on the

Glasgow Coma Scale. In contrast, among patients with some purposeful movements, favorable recovery is not uncommon. As with ICH, improvement is sometimes slow, and may continue well beyond 3 to 6 months.

Conclusion

ICH and SAH are both complex disorders, which commonly result in both neurological and systemic complications. Optimal management requires multidisciplinary collaboration. With ICH, efforts should focus especially on limiting early hematoma expansion and attenuating perihematomal edema. With SAH, clinicians should seek to prevent aneurysm rebleeding and limit both early and delayed ischemic injury. With both disorders, optimal neurocritical care emphasizes the timely recognition and treatment of potential causes of secondary brain injury. Accurate assessment of prognosis in patients with stupor and coma is not straightforward. Clinicians should communicate regularly with surrogate decision makers, rely on best available evidence, and acknowledge uncertainty when it exists.

Selected bibliography

1. Qureshi AI, Mendelow AD, Hanley DF. Intracerebral hemorrhage. *Lancet* 2009; **373**: 1632–44.
2. Xi G, Keep RF, Hoff JT. Mechanisms of brain injury after intracerebral hemorrhage. *Lancet Neurol* 2006; **5**: 53–63.
3. Demchuk AM, Dowlatshahi D, Rodriguez-Luna D, et al. Prediction of haematoma growth and outcome in patients with intracerebral haemorrhage using the CT-angiography spot sign (PREDICT): a prospective observational study. *Lancet Neurol* 2012; **11**: 307–14.
4. Kidwell CS, Chalela JA, Saver JL, et al. Comparison of MRI and CT for detection of acute intracerebral hemorrhage. *JAMA* 2004; **292**: 1823–30.
5. Mayer SA, Brun NC, Begtrup K, et al. Efficacy and safety of recombinant activated factor VII for acute intracerebral hemorrhage. *N Engl J Med* 2008; **358**: 2127–37.
6. Anderson CS, Huang Y, Want JG, et al. Intensive blood pressure reduction in acute cerebral haemorrhage trial (INTERACT): a randomised pilot trial. *Lancet* 2008; **7**: 391–99.

7. Morgenstern LB, Hemphill JC, Anderson C, et al. Guidelines for the management of spontaneous intracerebral hemorrhage. *Stroke* 2010; **41**: 2108–29.

8. Mendelow AD, Gregson BA, Fernandes HM, et al. Early surgery versus initial conservative treatment in patients with spontaneous supratentorial intracerebral haematomas in the international Surgical Trial in Intracerebral Hemorrhage (STICH): a randomised trial. *Lancet* 2005; **365**: 387–97.

9. Hemphill JC, Bonovich DC, Besmertis L, et al. The ICH score: a simple, reliable grading scale for intracerebral hemorrhage. *Stroke* 2001; **32**: 891–7.

10. Becker JK, Baxter AB, Cohen WA, et al. Withdrawal of support in intracerebral hemorrhage may lead to self-fulfilling prophecies. *Neurology* 2001; **56**: 766–72.

11. Suarez JI, Tarr RW, Selman WR. Aneurysmal subarachnoid hemorrhage. *N Engl J Med* 2006; **354**: 387–97.

12. Vergouwen MD, Vermeulen M, van Gijn J, et al. Definition of delayed cerebral ischemia after aneurysmal subarachnoid hemorrhage as an outcome event in clinical trials and observational studies: proposal of a multidisciplinary research group. *Stroke* 2010; **41**: 2391–5.

13. Sehba FA, Hou J, Pluta RM, Zhang JH. The importance of early brain injury after subarachnoid hemorrhage. *Prog Neurobiol* 2012; **97**: 14–37.

14. Rabinstein AA, Lanzino G, Wijdicks EFM. Multidisciplinary management and emerging therapeutic strategies in aneurysmal subarachnoid hemorrhage. *Lancet Neurol* 2010; **9**: 504–19.

15. Diringer MN, Bleck TP, Hemphill JC, et al. Critical care management of patients following aneurysmal subarachnoid hemorrhage: recommendations from the Neurocritical Care Society's multidisciplinary consensus conference. *Neurocrit Care* 2011; **15**: 211–40.

6

Prevention and Management of Poststroke Complications

Raid G. Ossi, MD

Department of Neurology, Mayo Clinic Florida, Jacksonville, Florida

Medical complications in stroke patients

Medical complications are common after stroke and can extend the length of hospital stay, worsen stroke outcome, limit recovery, impede rehabilitation, increase cost of care, and cause death. An odds ratio of in-hospital mortality of 3.62 (95% CI 2.80 to 4.68) was reported in a systematic review and meta-analysis of patients with poststroke infection [1]. Many complications are potentially preventable or treatable. There are certain factors that contribute to the likelihood of developing complications after stroke such as increasing age, co-morbidities, time since stroke, dehydration, malnutrition, prolonged immobilization, and dysphagia. Our aim as treating physicians is to influence these possible factors by interventions that may reduce the rate and severity of these complications (Table 6.1).

Venous thromboembolism

Venous thromboembolism (VTE), comprising pulmonary embolism (PE) and deep venous thrombosis (DVT), is a potentially fatal but preventable complication of stroke, and is associated with substantial morbidity and mortality. The highest incidence of DVT occurs between the second and seventh day post stroke. Without appropriate prophylaxis, up to 75% of patients with hemiplegia after stroke develop DVT, of these 20% are at risk of PE, which results in fatality in 1 to 2% of patients and causes 25% of early death following acute ischemic stroke. Fatal PE is unusual in the first week

and occurs most commonly 2 to 4 weeks following the stroke. Advanced age, immbolization after stroke, dehydration, and co-morbidities such as malignant diseases or clotting disorders increase the risk of DVT. The greatest clinical concern related to DVT is fatal PE. VTE is often asymptomatic and screening for its early detection is frequently performed by Duplex ultrasonography. Therapeutic options for DVT prophylaxis are summarized in Table 6.2.

> ★ **TIPS AND TRICKS**
>
> DVT prophylaxis should be routine for all patients with stroke. Pharmacologic prophylaxis (antithrombotic treatment) is contraindicated for 24 hours after intravenous rt-PA administration. Mechanical prophylaxis with sequential compression devices and antiembolic hose should be utilized in patients with contraindications to pharmacologic prophylaxis or until it can be safely initiated.

Recommendations support early mobilization after stroke as an effective measure to reduce the likelihood of DVT and other poststroke complications, thus potentially reducing the length of hospital stay. A randomized controlled pilot trial found an apparent reduction in severe complications and no increase in total complications with early mobilization after acute ischemic stroke [2].

Stroke, First Edition. Edited by Kevin M. Barrett and James F. Meschia.
© 2013 John Wiley & Sons, Ltd. Published 2013 by John Wiley & Sons, Ltd.

Table 6.1 Poststroke medical complications in hospitalized patients

Complication	Risk factors

Venous thromboembolism
   Deep venous thrombosis
   Pulmonary embolism
	Immobility
	Dehydration

Urinary tract complications
   Infections
   Voiding dysfunction
	Prolonged use of an indwelling catheter

Aspiration pneumonia	Impaired swallowing Immobility Nausea and vomiting

Nonbleeding complications of recombinant
   tissue plasminogen activator
   Lingual edema
   Anaphylactoid reactions
	Concomitant use of ACE inhibitors

Pressure sores and ulceration	Immobility Infrequent bed turning Dehydration
Falls	Immobility
Malnutrition	Impaired swallowing

Pain
   Shoulder pain
   Headache and musculoskeletal
	Reduced functional recovery and withdrawal from
	   rehabilitation programs
	Overuse, over-stretching, and poor resting postures

Miscellaneous medical complications
   Cardiac complications
   Gastrointestinal complications
	Cardiac: co-morbid cardiac disease
	Gastrointestinal: older age, stroke severity,
	   inactivity, and type of food

Neuropsychiatric disturbances Delirium	Brain ischemia Infections Electrolyte disturbances

Table 6.2 Prophylaxis for venous thromboembolism

Method	Comment
Early mobilization	Close monitoring of blood pressure and neurological status is needed, because hemodynamically unstable patients or those with fluctuating symptoms cannot be safely mobilized. Patients treated with thrombolytics are routinely kept on bed rest for the first 24 hours while in intensive care units.

Mechanical compressive devices
   Graduated compression
     stockings
   Intermittent pneumatic
     compression devices
	Useful for prophylaxis in those with contraindications to antithrombotic therapy and in the first 24 hours post-thrombolysis. Caution is advised to patients with severe peripheral arterial disease, peripheral neuropathy, or cognitive impairment.

Unfractionated heparin	Contraindicated in the first 24 hours after intravenous recombinant tissue plasminogen activator. Effective in reducing incidence of deep venous thrombosis/pulmonary embolism. Does not require monitoring. Hemorrhage risk may be concerning in patients with large strokes or history of systemic bleeding.
Low-molecular-weight heparins	Contraindicated in the first 24 hours after intravenous recombinant tissue plasminogen activator. Requires less frequent dosing than unfractionated heparin. Risk: benefit ratio compared with unfractionated heparin is unclear. Majority of benefit is observed in preventing asymptomatic venous thrombosis.

However, hemodynamically unstable patients or those with fluctuating symptoms cannot be safely mobilized, because orthostatic hypotension may cause watershed infarction. Also, patients treated with thrombolytics are routinely kept on bed rest for the first 24 hours while in the intensive care unit for fear that falls could lead to severe bleeding complications.

Several mechanical compressive devices are available for DVT prophylaxis. Tight-fitting knee-high or thigh-high antiembolic stockings reduce venous stasis in the leg, although some patients find them uncomfortable and difficult to tolerate. They should be used with caution in patients with significant peripheral arterial disease to avoid compromise of distal circulation. Pneumatic compression devices exert a pumping action that attempts to simulate the normal muscular contraction used to move dependent venous blood against gravity. Pneumatic compression devices may increase the risk of falls by being an unintended two-point restraint system. Use of bed alarms may reduce risk of falls when using these devices. Although randomized clinical trial evidence has not demonstrated relative efficacy of graduated compression stockings to reduce the risk of DVT after acute stroke, mechanical compressive devices are commonly used for prophylaxis in those with contraindications to antithrombotic therapy and in patients with hemorrhagic infarcts.

The subcutaneous administration of unfractionated heparin (UFH) and low-molecular-weight heparin (LMWH) is recommended for treatment of immobilized patients and this has been demonstrated to reduce the risk of VTE events after stroke. The ideal timing for starting these medications has not been established given concerns for intracranial or systemic hemorrhage, particularly in patients with large ischemic stroke [3]. A meta-analysis of controlled studies in patients with hemorrhagic stroke found early anticoagulation is associated with a significant reduction in PE and a nonsignificant reduction in mortality. This was balanced by a nonsignificant increase in hematoma enlargement [4]. In practice, initiation of anticoagulation for DVT prophylaxis is often delayed for 2 to 3 days after diagnosis in patients with intracerebral hemorrhage. In patients with significant hemorrhagic transformation, anticoagulation should be deferred until bleeding has stabilized.

⚠ CAUTION

Anticoagulant and antiplatelet agents should not be used for 24 hours after administration of recombinant tissue plasminogen activator (rt-PA).

EVIDENCE AT A GLANCE

The results of pooled analyses suggest that low-dose LMWH have the best benefit/risk ratio in patients with acute ischemic stroke by decreasing the risk of both DVT and pulmonary embolism, without a clear increase in intracranial or extracranial hemorrhage [5]. The Prevention of Venous Thromboembolism after acute Ischemic Stroke With LMWH (PREVAIL) trial, involving 1762 ischemic stroke patients, demonstrated that enoxaparin (40 mg daily) was superior to UFH (5000 U every 12 hours) in preventing VTE in patients with ischemic stroke and was associated with a small but significant increase in extracranial hemorrhage rates; this was mainly nonfatal gastrointestinal bleeding [6]. A secondary analysis of PREVAIL showed that the clinical benefits of VTE prophylaxis were not associated with poorer long-term neurological outcomes or increased rates of symptomatic intracranial hemorrhage compared with UFH [7].

Urinary tract complications

Urinary tract complications include urinary tract infection (UTI) and bladder dysfunction. Poststroke UTI is common during the first 5 days after hospital admission. UTI is associated with poorer outcomes, increased likelihood of a decline in neurological status during hospitalization, and increased length of hospital stay. Most UTIs are associated with use of indwelling bladder catheters for urinary retention or incontinence after stroke. Prolonged use of bladder catheters is discouraged because of their association with infection; intermittent bladder catheterization may be a safer alternative. Bladder catheterization for routine monitoring of urine output, urinary incontinence, and nursing convenience should be avoided when possible.

★ TIPS AND TRICKS

Foley catheter placement indications include (but not limited to):

- acute retention or obstruction;
- the need for accurate measurement of urinary output in critically ill patients;
- patients requiring prolonged immobilization.

Bladder dysfunction in the forms of urinary incontinence and retention are common after stroke. Pharmacological therapy with anticholinergic medications may help speed the return of bladder function; however, these agents should be avoided given the potential for adverse cognitive effects. Prophylactic administration of antibiotics for UTI is not recommended. The use of preventive antibiotics in stroke, and the effect of this therapy on antibiotic resistance, is currently under investigation in a large randomized clinical trial [8]. Routine urinalysis obtained as part of a fever evaluation will identify the majority of urinary tract infections. Prompt antibiotic treatment for documented UTI minimizes the risk of bacteremia or sepsis; acidification of urine also may lessen the risk of infection.

Aspiration pneumonia

Pneumonia is the most common poststroke infection, with a rate of 10%. Pneumonia after stroke is associated with a significantly increased cost of hospitalization and likelihood of extended care requirements upon discharge. Severely affected stroke patients are often immobile, with impaired swallowing, poor cough, and nausea or vomiting, which may increase the risk of aspiration pneumonia. However, chest infection may develop in patients without clinically apparent aspiration.

Ventilator-associated pneumonia (VAP) is a common infection in critically ill patients that is associated with poor clinical and economic outcomes. VAP is preventable and many practices have been demonstrated to reduce the incidence of VAP and its associated burden of illness. The Institute for Healthcare Improvement developed the "Ventilator Bundle" consisting of four evidence-based practices to improve outcomes of patients requiring mechanical ventilation; the components are as follows: (1) elevation of the head of the bed to 35 to 45°; (2) daily "sedation vacation" and daily assessment of readiness to extubate; (3) peptic ulcer disease prophylaxis; and (4) DVT prophylaxis [9].

★ TIPS AND TRICKS

General measures to help lower the risk of aspiration pneumonia:

- Protection of the airway, airway suction, and aggressive pulmonary toilet.
- Elevation of the head of bed to 45°. When this is not possible, attempts to raise the head of the bed as much as possible should be considered.
- Appropriate evaluation of swallowing function and modification of oral intake. A 3-ounce water swallow test performed at the bedside is a useful screening tool.
- Exercise and encouragement to take deep breaths, and incentive spirometry can facilitate air movement and prevent atelectasis at the lung bases.
- Mobilization and frequent changes in position.
- Use measures to treat nausea to prevent vomiting.

Prompt antibiotic therapy is warranted in patients with radiographically confirmed chest infection and in those where the clinical suspicion is high. Empiric coverage for both aerobic and anaerobic pathogens should be used to treat patients with presumed aspiration until results of cultures and sensitivities are available.

✋ CAUTION

- Prophylactic administration of antibiotics for pneumonia is not recommended.
- The appearance of fever after stroke should prompt a search for pneumonia and appropriate antibiotic therapy should be administered.

Nonbleeding complications of recombinant tissue plasminogen activator

Anaphylaxis after treatment with recombinant tissue plasminogen activator (rt-PA) for acute ischemic stroke is an uncommon complication.

The risk of anaphylaxis is increased in patients treated with angiotensin converting enzyme (ACE) inhibitors. Orolingual angioedema and anaphylaxis up to 2 hours after intravenous infusion of rt-PA have been reported. Patients who suffer life-threatening angioedema, laryngospasm, and hypotension should be immediately treated with antihistamines, intravenous corticosteroids, epi-nephrine, and discontinuation of the rt-PA infusion as clinically indicated.

★ TIPS AND TRICKS

- Orolingual edema is generally a unilateral phenomenon limited to the lips and tongue contralateral to the affected hemisphere.
- Posterior extension of edema to the oropharynx may lead to life-threatening upper airway obstruction – careful examination of the tongue and oropharynx of patients receiving rt-PA, especially those taking ACE inhibitors, is recommended.
- Swelling typically develops gradually over several hours; a period of observation may be appropriate to ensure the airway is not threatened.

Pressure sores and ulceration

Pressure sores and ulcerations are preventable com-plications that impose a huge cost to the health-care system. Pressure ulcers usually develop over a bony prominence as a result of sustained pressure, partic-ularly in those that are immobilized and malnour-ished. Successful prevention is a continuous process that often requires an multidisciplinary team. Early mobilization of neurologically stable patients can help reduce the risk of pressure sores and ulcera-tion. For patients who can not be safely mobilized, routine assessment for skin breakdown, particularly in dependent areas, is recommended. Frequent turning, every 2 hours, can help minimize the risk of decubitus ulcers. Skin should be kept dry and free of moisture, particularly in patients with urinary incontinence. In some situations, oscillating mattress systems may be necessary to minimize prolonged pressure on susceptible areas (sacrum, greater trochanter). Antibiotics and debridement may be necessary in cases of severe skin breakdown.

Falls

Patients with stroke are at high risk for falls relative to other hospitalized patients. A retrospective study including patients admitted to 23 hospitals found an incidence of falls of 8.9% per 1000 patients per day [10]. Another retrospective cohort study of patients with ischemic stroke found that 5% of patients with an ischemic stroke fell during the acute inpatient hospitalization [11]. Putative risk factors include cognitive, motor, sensory, balance impairment, hemineglect, polypharmacy, and urinary inconti-nence. Fall prevention should be an important part of initial mobilization, and identifying patients at highest risk is necessary to target fall prevention measures appropriately. Nurses play an important role in minimizing falls by assessing risk of falls at the time of admission, putting commonly needed items within arm's reach, keeping the bed in a low position, and encouraging the patient to ask for assistance.

The use of physical restraints to prevent falls should be avoided if possible. Observational studies of restraint reduction programs showed a significant reduction in the rates of injurious falls even though the rates of minor falls increased or remained unchanged. Physical restraints are well docu-mented by research and several US government and health-care quality groups to cause death, significant injury, and iatrogenic complications, yet this practice continues in hospitals and nursing homes. The Joint Commission on Accreditation of Healthcare Organizations (JCAHO) has tracked death and injury from restraints as sentinel events since 1995. Negative consequences associated with physical restraints may be grouped into: (1) physical iatrogenic outcomes: increased risk for falling, pressure ulcers, incontinence, muscle decondition-ing, and acute functional decline, serious injuries: hip fracture, head trauma; and (2) psychological, behavioral combativeness, aggression, increased disorientation, regression, and dependency [12]. A randomized controlled trial [13] concluded that access to a bed-chair pressure sensor device nei-ther reduced the use of physical restraints nor improved the clinical outcomes of older patients with perceived fall risk. The provision of bed-chair pressure sensors may only be effective in reducing physical restraints when it is combined with an organized physical restraint reduction program.

★ TIPS AND TRICKS

Measures to prevent poststroke falls in acute hospital setting:

- use of assistive walking devices;
- motion detectors;
- bed alarms;
- use of convex mirrors to enable nursing staff to view hallways from nursing stations;
- nonslip footwear for patients;
- minimal use of sedative medications.

Malnutrition

Patients that cannot safely receive oral intake because of dysphagia or decreased level of consciousness after stroke are at increased risk of dehydration, malnutrition, and death. Malnutrition is prevalent in patients with three or more strokes, National Institutes of Health Stroke Scale (NIHSS) scores ≥15, and modified Rankin scale scores of 4–5. Malnutrition risk is also associated with poststroke depression, lack of family support, and lack of early rehabilitation. A valid assessment of swallowing function should be performed before the patient is cleared for oral intake. Indicators of dysphagia such as an abnormal gag reflex, impaired voluntary cough, dysphonia, incomplete orolabial closure, and cranial nerve palsies should be assessed routinely. There are other features that place stroke patients at highest risk for dysphagia, such as a brain stem stroke, impaired consciousness, slurred speech, hoarse voice, and a wet voice.

★ TIPS AND TRICKS

The 3-oz water swallow test:

- The test is performed at the bedside and is a useful and sensitive screening tool for patients without high-risk features.
- The patient is given 3 oz (≈ 90 mL) of water in a cup and asked to drink without interruption. If the patient is able to complete the task without a cough or change in voice quality, the patient can be cleared for "oral intake."
- Coughing or change in voice quality up to 1 minute after drinking warrants NPO status until a formal evaluation by a speech pathologist has been completed.

Patients who can not safely take food or liquids orally may require a nasogastric or nasoduodenal tube to provide feedings and administration of medications. These measures, however, do not eliminate the risk of aspiration pneumonia. Many patients will demonstrate early improvement of their swallowing mechanism in the days following stroke, thus repeated assessment and documentation of swallowing function will assist in the removal of parenteral feeding tubes as soon as possible. A percutaneous endoscopic gastrostomy (PEG) tube is often used when the need for a parenteral feeding tube is anticipated to be longer than 7 days. PEG tubes are more comfortable than tubes inserted in the nose, facilitate mobilization, and generally require less care. Disadvantages include dislodging of the tube, risk of bleeding at the time of insertion in patients treated with antithrombotic medications, and peritonitis. The FOOD Trial Collaboration studies found no benefit for early placement of PEG tubes after stroke [14].

EVIDENCE AT A GLANCE

The FOOD Trial Collaboration conducted the FOOD trials which consist of three pragmatic multicenter randomized controlled trials, two of which included dysphagic stroke patients. In one trial, patients enrolled within 7 days of admission were randomly allocated to early enteral tube feeding or no tube feeding for more than 7 days (early versus avoid). In the other, patients were allocated PEG or nasogastric feeding. The primary outcome was death or poor outcome at 6 months. These results suggest that early tube feeding may reduce case fatality, but increased the proportion of patients surviving with poor outcomes. The data do not support a policy of early initiation of PEG feeding in stroke patients with dysphagia.

Daily calorie counts can help prevent malnutrition during an acute hospitalization. Fluid balance should be monitored, and intravenous normal saline (0.9% NaCl) should be used to maintain adequate volume status.

⚠ CAUTION

In patients with restricted or limited oral fluid intake, hypotonic saline should be avoided, as it may cause osmotic shifts of free water from the extracellular to the intracellular compartment and exacerbate peri-infarct edema.

Pain

Shoulder pain in a paretic limb is a common complication in patients with significant proximal arm weakness. Poststroke pain is multifactorial in origin, the most common noncentral and musculoskeletal etiologies of hemiplegic shoulder pain include adhesive capsulitis, subluxation, and rotator cuff pathologies. Hemiplegic shoulder pain is associated with reduction in functional use of the arm, interference with rehabilitation, and increased length of hospitalization. Functional electrical stimulation, positioning programs, external shoulder support devices, and intra-articular steroid injections have been used with variable degrees of success to reduce shoulder discomfort.

Headache and musculoskeletal pains involving the cervical or lumbar spine, hip, knee, and ankle are common after stroke and during rehabilitation. Anti-inflammatory medications and the discretionary use of orthotic devices may minimize these complications.

Miscellaneous medical complications

Cardiac complications

Many patients with stroke have co-morbid cardiac disease and require surveillance for cardiac arrhythmias and myocardial ischemia. As part of the initial stroke assessment, a standard 12-lead ECG and continuous telemetry to capture a paroxysmal arrhythmia are recommended. Patients with symptoms of cardiac disease or ST-segment changes on ECG should have serial cardiac enzymes to exclude concurrent myocardial ischemia. Many patients with acute stroke will have echocardiography, which can assist in identifying structural heart disease.

Gastrointestinal (GI) complications

Bleeding, constipation, fecal impaction, and diarrhea are common GI complications. GI bleeding may occur in the acute stroke setting with older

patients those with greater stroke severity at highest risk. In patients who are unable to safely take food or liquids by mouth, it is reasonable to use proton-pump inhibitors and H2-antagonists as a GI prophylaxis, even though the current guidelines do not recommend routine use of GI prophylaxis for all patients with stroke. A word of caution is appropriate regarding certain proton pump inhibitors, as these may reduce the antiplatelet effects of clopidogrel. In stroke patients with constipation associated with rectal impaction with overflow, suppositories rather than increased doses of laxatives are recommended. Whereas in stroke patients with constipation and weak anal sphincters, the advice is to use a bulking agent rather than a stool softener to avoid anal leakage. Some feedings administered via a percutaneous endoscopic gastrostomy tube or nasogastric tube may cause osmotic gradients that lead to diarrhea.

Neuropsychiatric disturbances

Numerous emotional and behavioral disorders occur following stroke. Depression being the most common; delirium, emotional lability, anxiety, mania, and apathy are well recognized neuropsychiatric complications of stroke.

Delirium (acute confusional state)

Delirium poses a common and serious complication in hospitalized elderly patients. The prevalence of delirium in the acute setting of stroke varies from 13 to 48%. Delirium is a strong predictor of adverse outcomes, longer in-patient stay, and increased risk of mortality; in an observational study, delirium was found to be an independent predictor of inpatient mortality (30.4 versus 1.7%, $P <0.001$) [15].

Independent risk factors for poststroke delirium include a left-sided stroke, intracerebral hemorrhage, cardioembolic stroke; total anterior circulation infarction, older age, pre-existing cognitive impairment, dysphagia, neglect, vision field loss, lower blood pressure, and lower Glasgow Coma Scale scores. Patients with delirium are also more likely to have medical complications such as urinary tract infection, urinary or fecal incontinence, and metabolic disorders.

Delirium is often unrecognized, perhaps because it may develop rapidly and fluctuates between a hyperactive and hypoactive form. Common clinical features of delirium include acute onset of altered level of consciousness, inattention, disorganized thinking, with disturbances in orientation, memory, perception and behavior; hallucinations, paratonia, and asterexis may accompany delirium. The causative factors should be aggressively identified and addressed given the high morbidity and mortality associated with delirium. To identify cases of delirium at an early stage after stroke, delirium screening on admission should be considered and be incorporated into the initial stroke assessments.

> ⭐ **TIPS AND TRICKS**
>
> Delirium screening on admission should be considered and be incorporated into the initial stroke assessments.

There are several formal tools that can be effective for delirium screening. The Confusion Assessment Method (CAM), developed in 1990, is sensitive, specific, reliable, and easy to use. CAM could be used by general health professionals to identify delirium rapidly and accurately. The CAM instrument, which can be completed in less than 5 minutes, consists of nine operationalized criteria from the Diagnostic and Statistical Manual of Mental Disorders (DSM-III-R). The CAM algorithm for diagnosis of delirium is based on four features: (1) acute onset and fluctuating course; (2) inattention; (3) disorganized thinking; and (4) altered level of consciousness. The CAM algorithm for diagnosis of delirium required the presence of both the first and the second criteria and either the third or the fourth criterion.

The Delirium Rating Scale (DRS) is a 10-item symptom severity rating scale based on DSM-III criteria that is intended for use by clinicians with psychiatric training. Each item has specific descriptors that can be scored from 0 to a maximum of 2, 3, or 4 points, depending on the 10 items of scale: temporal onset, perceptual disturbances, hallucinations, delusions, psychomotor disturbance, cognitive status, physical disorder, sleep–wake disturbance, lability of mood, and variability of symptoms. Individual item scores are summed to generate a 32-point scale. A score greater or equal to 10 is conventionally used to diagnose delirium. Unlike the CAM, which only assesses if delirium is present, the DRS also includes a measure of delirium severity.

The Mini Mental State Examination (MMSE) is a routinely used bedside test that can identify stroke patients at risk of developing delirium. It is a brief 30-point questionnaire test that is used to screen for cognitive impairment. MMSE scores are used to classify patients with severe (<10 points), moderate (10–20 points), mild (21–25 points), or no (26–30 points) cognitive impairment. MMSE score is influenced by patients' educational background, language, mood, and sensory/motor function, which render it potentially challenging to interpret in the acute stroke setting; nonetheless, MMSE scores <10 points are associated with poststroke delirium [15]. The same study concluded that the CAM is equivalent to the DRS in the detection of delirium poststroke, and that the MMSE should be avoided when specifically assessing patients for delirium in the acute stroke setting.

Following screening for delirium in an acute stroke setting, the possible causative factor should be sought, identified, and managed accordingly; electrolyte disturbances, signs and symptoms of an accompanying infection, fever, high leukocyte count, and a high sedimentation rate should be assessed.

Neurological complications in stroke patients

Neurological complications are less frequent than medical complications and typically occur earlier after acute stroke presentation. Neurological complications can adversely affect short- and long-term outcomes. The most frequent neurological complications of stroke are listed in Table 6.3.

Some of these complications can be prevented; others can be properly managed to reduce their negative effects on outcomes.

Table 6.3 Poststroke neurological complications in hospitalized patients

Cerebral edema
Hemorrhagic transformation
Seizures
Miscellaneous neurological complications
Headache
Sleep disorders
Sleep-disordered breathing

Cerebral edema

Mass effect due to cerebral edema may complicate proximal anterior circulation occlusions and cerebellar infarction. Cerebral edema with neurological deterioration may occur as early as 48 to 72 hours after ischemic stroke onset. Space-occupying mass effect is the leading cause of mortality in the first week following large territorial infarctions.

> ### ⚗ SCIENCE REVISITED
>
> *Pathophysiology of brain edema*: the primary cause of brain edema is cellular ionic imbalance due to energy depletion caused by ischemia. Two types of edema (cytotoxic and vasogenic) occur in patients with ischemic stroke. Cytotoxic edema is characterized by the translocation of interstitial water into the intracellular compartment and occurs early, when the blood–brain barrier is still intact. At the late stage of stroke, the blood–brain barrier is compromised, causing vasogenic edema, characterized by fluid movement from vascular to extravascular spaces. Vasogenic edema leads to an expansion of brain volume with increased intracranial pressure, herniation, and exacerbation of ischemia. Differentiation of cytotoxic and vasogenic brain edema in the clinical setting is important for diagnostic and therapeutic purposes because cytotoxic edema is unresponsive to traditional pharmacological treatment. Recent advances in MRI can differentiate cytotoxic and vasogenic edema. Cytotoxic edema causes a reduction in the diffusion of water molecules and demonstrates increased signal intensity on diffusion-weighted MRI. Vasogenic edema causes increased water in brain tissues, which can appear on conventional T2-weighted images and fluid-attenuated inversion recovery (FLAIR) sequences.

The development of cerebral edema within 24 hours of stroke with altered consciousness, third nerve palsy, or other signs of cerebral herniation has been termed malignant middle cerebral artery (MCA) infarction (MMI). Large ischemic strokes involving the MCA territory often cause conjugate gaze preference, dense hemiplegia, dense hemi-sensory disturbance, homonymous hemianopia, and aphasia or hemispatial neglect, depending on whether the dominant or nondominant hemisphere is involved. Additional symptoms and signs may suggest the development of space-occupying edema including headache, vomiting, papilledema, deteriorating neurological function, and reduced level of consciousness. The additional manifestations evolving from MMI are largely because of focal edema and displacement of the brain, rather than a global increase in intracranial pressure. Patients under the age of 50 years are generally at higher risk owing to the absence of cerebral atrophy. Predictors of MMI have the potential to influence clinical management decisions. Coma at the time of initial clinical evaluation and severe neurological deficit as measured by an NIHSS >20 are associated with fatal cerebral edema. CT scan findings, such as an extensive zone of early ischemia (e.g. involving >50% of the MCA territory), the presence of a hyperdense MCA sign, and carotid terminus occlusion are also predictors. Early signs on noncontrast head CT predictive of a MMI include lateral anteroseptal shift of ≥5 mm, lateral pineal shift of ≥2 mm, hydrocephalus, temporal lobe infarction, and the presence of other vascular territory infarction (anterior cerebral artery and/or posterior cerebral artery territories). Diffusion-weighted imaging (DWI) can also useful for prediction of MMI within the first 6 hours of stroke.

Cerebellar infarction can result in brainstem compression and obstructive hydrocephalus when significant edema develops within the restricted confines of the posterior fossa. Cerebellar edema usually peaks on the third day after the infarction, however it may occur earlier or later. Rapid clinical deterioration can occur because of obstructive hydrocephalus, but it can also occur due to sudden apnea or cardiac arrhythmia associated with brainstem compression.

Reliable prediction of those at highest risk to develop life-threatening cerebral edema has proven difficult. Clinical variables associated with increased risk include a history of hypertension or heart failure and presence of leukocytosis. A retrospective series that included autopsy data found younger age, female gender, absence of prior stroke history, higher heart weight, carotid artery occlusion, and an

Table 6.4 Selected medical therapy for cerebral edema

Therapy	Comments
Mannitol	Mechanism: osmotic agent facilitates movement of free water from the interstitial/intracellular compartment across intact blood–brain barrier (i.e. osmotic diuresis). May decrease blood viscosity. Initial bolus 20% mannitol; 1 g/kg. Maintenance regimens use 0.5 or 0.25 g/kg every 4–6 h titrated to achieve serum osmolality between 310 and 320 mOsm/L.
Hypertonic saline	Mechanism: osmotic agent expands intravascular volume versus diuretic effect of mannitol. Potential complications include hypernatremia, congestive heart failure, and pulmonary edema. Concentrations range from 3 to 23.4% saline with various bolus and continuous dosing regimens. Central venous access needed for administration of higher concentrations.
Barbiturates	Mechanism: decreases cerebral metabolism with reduction of cerebral blood flow. Severe complications include hypotension (with impaired cerebral perfusion pressure), hepatic dysfunction, and increased risk of infection. Limited and short-lasting benefit with potential for severe complications.
Glycerol	Mechanism: potent hypertonic agent. The drug rapidly lowers intracranial pressure within 30 minutes following oral or intravenous dose. The main effect of glycerin results from its osmotic dehydrating effects, although other mechanisms have been postulated for its effect in lowering intracranial pressure. These include an increase in blood flow to ischemic areas, decreases in serum free fatty acids, and increases in synthesis of glycerides in the brain. Glycerol is usually administered intravenously over 1 hour in a dose of 250 mL 4–6 times a day. During administration, blood osmolarity should be monitored and maintained at approximately 300–320 mOsm/L.
Hyperventilation	Mechanism: induces cerebral vasoconstriction with reduction of cerebral blood flow and volume. Duration of benefit is limited (i.e. hours). May reduce blood flow to near ischemic levels. Potential for rebound vasodilatation and increasing edema and intracranial pressure. Partial pressure of carbon dioxide, arterial ($Paco_2$) often targeted to 30 mmHg.
Elevated head position 30°	Mechanism: increases venous outflow with reduction of cranial venous hydrostatic pressure and volume. May reduce cerebral perfusion pressure due to decreased mean arterial pressure.

abnormal ipsilateral circle of Willis were more frequent in patients who developed brain swelling and herniation.

The optimal nonsurgical treatment of cerebral edema remains controversial. Conventional medical approaches to the treatment of cerebral edema and elevated intracranial pressure are listed in Table 6.4.

These strategies are often employed empirically or as a temporizing measure to a more definitive therapy to control space-occupying mass effect such as decompressive hemicraniectomy. Consistent evidence supporting a beneficial effect on functional outcomes for these interventions is lacking.

★ **TIPS AND TRICKS**

- Restriction of free water may reduce the likelihood of a hypo-osmolar state that could potentially worsen edema.
- Hypoxemia, hypercarbia, and hyperthermia may worsen cerebral edema and should be managed aggressively.
- The head of the bed can be elevated to 20–30° to reduce intracranial pressure (ICP) by promoting venous outflow.

The rationale behind the use of osmotic agents for raised ICP is to create an osmotic gradient across the blood–brain barrier, drawing water from the interstitial and intracellular space to the intravascular space. When the blood–brain barrier is compromised, rebound cerebral edema and progressive herniation may develop with the use of osmotic agents. Mannitol, hypertonic saline, and glycerol are the most frequently used osmotic agents; prospective data surrounding their use for space-occupying edema in cerebral infarction are lacking; moreover, no evidence indicates that hyperventilation, corticosteroids in conventional or large doses, furosemide, mannitol, or glycerol or other measures that reduce ICP improve outcome in patients with ischemic brain stroke.

⚓ CAUTION

- Corticosteroids (in conventional or large doses) are not recommended for treatment of cerebral edema and increased intracranial pressure complicating ischemic stroke.
- Antihypertensive agents, particularly those that cause cerebral venodilatation, such as sodium nitroprusside and hydralazine, should be avoided given the theoretical risk of exacerbating increases in ICP.
- Hyperventilation is generally not recommended because it causes cerebral vasoconstriction, potentially exacerbating ischemic injury.

Medical management of malignant MCA infarction is generally ineffective, with conservative treatment carrying a mortality rate of about 80%.

EVIDENCE AT A GLANCE

A pooled analysis of three European randomized, controlled trials (Decompressive Craniectomy for Malignant Middle Cerebral Artery Infarction (DECIMAL), Decompressive Surgery for the Treatment of Malignant Infarction of the Middle Cerebral Artery (DESTINY), and Hemicraniectomy After Middle Cerebral Artery Infarction with Life-Threatening Edema Trial (HAMLET)), demonstrated that hemicraniectomy reduces mortality and improves favorable functional outcome when performed within 48 hours of stroke onset [16].

Hemicraniectomy and duraplasty have been used as definitive therapy for life-threatening space-occupying edema resulting from MMI. Decompressive surgery can create a space for the swollen brain to move out of the cranial cavity rather than compressing critical brainstem structures. Results from case series demonstrate improved outcomes with the use of ventriculostomy and suboccipital craniectomy for patients with progressive clinical deterioration due to massive cerebellar infarction. Patients with cerebellar hemorrhage who are deteriorating neurologically or who have brainstem compression and/or hydrocephalus from ventricular obstruction should undergo surgical removal of the hemorrhage as soon as possible (Class 1; Level of Evidence B). Initial treatment of these patients with ventricular drainage alone rather than surgical evacuation is not recommended (Class III; Level of Evidence C) [17].

Hemorrhagic transformation

Hemorrhagic transformation (HT) of acute ischemic stroke is an important complication of thrombolysis and antithrombotic therapy, particularly anticoagulation. Not every HT carries the same clinical consequence. HT can also occur spontaneously after stroke in patients who do not receive thrombolysis. On close inspection, histopathologic examination of cerebral infarction often identifies some degree of petechial hemorrhage. However, this petechial blood is usually not associated with neurological deterioration. In the National Institute of Neurological Disorders and Stroke (NINDS) rt-PA study, symptomatic intracranial hemorrhage was defined as neurologic deterioration with computed tomography evidence of intracranial hemorrhage. Radiographically, the prevalence of spontaneous HT was 8.5% in untreated patients. HT accompanied by neurologic deterioration or frank hematoma formation occurs in 1.5%. The frequency is higher in patients treated with antithrombotic or thrombolytic drugs. Larger infarct size with mass effect and advanced patient age (>70 years) may be predisposing factors. A classification scheme for hemorrhagic transformation was used in the ECASS II trial and has subsequently gained acceptance as a classification scheme used in other research [18]. This system differentiates hemorrhagic infarction from parenchymal hematoma (PH). HT1 is a hemorrhagic infarct with petechiae along the margins of infarction. HT2 is a hemorrhagic infarct with more confluent petechiae, but no mass effect. PH1 is a PH in ≤30% of the infarct with no or slight mass effect, and PH2 is a PH in >30% of the infarct with substantial mass effect. It is the PH2 type of hemorrhage that independently predicts poor outcomes.

The best methods for preventing bleeding complications are careful selection of suitable patients for thrombolytic therapy and scrupulous care, especially frequent neurological observation and monitoring of the patients with early treatment of arterial hypertension [3]. There is no single intervention that has been studied in a rigorous prospective fashion, and most management recommendations are empirical or based on expert consensus.

⚡ CAUTION

The use of anticoagulants and antiplatelet agents should be delayed for 24 hours after treating cerebral infarction with intravenous tissue plasminogen activator.

Many patients with evidence of HT are managed conservatively with short-term discontinuation of antithrombotic agents and careful control of arterial blood pressure. Management of patients with symptomatic intracranial hemorrhage depends on the amount of bleeding and its symptoms, and may include clot evacuation in a deteriorating patient owing to hematoma-related mass effect to prevent herniation.

★ TIPS AND TRICKS

- Hyperglycemia is associated with HT, and thus treatment of hyperglycemia may reduce the risk of hemorrhagic transformation.
- Body temperature at 24 hours post-thrombolysis tends to be higher in patients with HT. As hyperthermia carries a poor prognosis in acute stroke, treating fevers may be beneficial in patients with HT.

Seizures

Seizures in stroke patients are a common complication and adversely affect neurological outcome. Seizures can occur early after the onset of ischemic stroke or can be a late complication. Early seizures are usually defined as those that occur within 1 or 2 weeks after stroke. The reported frequency of early seizures during the first days of stroke ranges from 2 to 23%, late seizures vary from 3 to 67%, depending on the study cohort [3]. Epilepsy (recurrent seizures) develops in 2.5–4% of patients. Patients who develop seizures within 14 days after stroke have poor prognosis with a high in-hospital mortality rate; however, they have a significantly lower rate of recurrent seizures compared to patients with late seizures. Status epilepticus may develop in a small proportion of patients with poststroke seizures, and negatively affects outcomes and mortality.

SCIENCE REVISITED

Pathophysiology of early poststroke seizures: in the first few days following an ischemic brain lesion, cellular biochemical dysfunction can lead to cortical excitability and seizure activity. Acute ischemia and anoxia during a stroke lead to massive release of the excitatory amino acid neurotransmitter glutamate, causing excessive activation of postsynaptic glutamate receptors believed to be the major cause of neuronal injury in stroke. Glutamate receptor activation has been strongly associated with epileptogenesis.

In a large population-based study, 3.1% of patients had seizures in the first 24 hours after stroke onset [19]. Risk factors for poststroke seizures include: large cortical infarcts, involvement of multiple sites, embolic stroke, stroke severity, size of the infarct, decreased consciousness, and hemodynamic and metabolic disturbance. Seizures occur more often in patients with dural sinus thrombosis than in patients with arterial stroke and might be the initial form of presentation in dural sinus thrombosis.

★ TIPS AND TRICKS

- Seizures rarely occur during thrombolysis and may, in the absence of intracerebral hemorrhage, be a favorable prognostic sign reflecting reperfusion. Seizures can be a manifestation of cerebral reperfusion injury after administration of rt-PA for acute ischemic stroke.
- Nonconvulsive seizures, which are difficult to detect clinically because

electroencephalography is needed for diagnosis, might account for neurological deterioration in some cases.
- Prophylactic administration of anticonvulsants to patients after stroke is not recommended.

Anticonvulsant therapy should be initiated in patients with witnessed or suspected poststroke seizures. In early onset seizures and status epilepticus, intravenous benzodiazepines are the first choice, eventually followed by phenytoin, sodium valproate, or carbamazepine. The optimal duration of therapy has not been established.

⚠ CAUTION

The choice of an anticonvulsant drug should be guided by the individual characteristics of each patient. Most first-generation anticonvulsant drugs, particularly phenytoin, might not be the optimal choice in stroke patients, and special consideration should be given to the possible interaction with anticoagulants and salicylates, side-effects, and adverse effects on poststroke recovery. New generation anticonvulsants, such as lamotrigine, gabapentin, and levetiracetam might be appropriate first-line treatments for poststroke seizures in elderly patients or patients with concurrent medical co-morbidities and medications.

Miscellaneous neurological complications

Headache

Headache is reported variably after stroke. After ischemic stroke, headache is typically ipsilateral to the cerebral infarction. Supratentorial lesions can be associated with headache in the anterior half of the head, presumably related to shared innervation by the ophthalmic division of the trigeminal nerve. Infratentorial lesions are associated with headache in the posterior half of the head. Ischemic stroke can cause a migraine syndrome in patients who previously did not have a history of migraine or can precipitate a migraine attack in patients predisposed to migraine.

EVIDENCE AT A GLANCE

The Lausanne Stroke Registry included 2506 patients with first ever stroke and patients were questioned about headache within 12 hours of symptom onset. In this registry, 18% of patients reported headache: 14% with anterior circulation stroke and 29% with posterior circulation stroke ($P<0.001$). Headache was reported by 16% of the patients with infarct and 36% of those with hemorrhage ($P<0.001$). The prevalence of headache was 9% with lacunar infarct, 15% with middle cerebral artery territory infarct, 37% with infratentorial hemorrhage, and 36% with supratentorial hemorrhage. The most common topography of pain was frontal (41%), followed by diffuse headache (27%; $P<0.001$). Diffuse (41%) or occipital (30%) headache was particularly frequent with posterior circulation stroke, whereas frontal headache was associated with anterior circulation stroke (51%; $P<0.001$) [20].

SCIENCE REVISITED

Pain-sensitive structures include the main trunks of the dural arteries, the intracranial segment of the internal carotid artery, the middle cerebral artery (proximal 1–2 cm), proximal anterior cerebral artery (from its origin to 1 cm beyond the genu of the corpus callosum), 1 to 2 cm of the intracranial vertebral artery, anterior inferior cerebellar artery, posterior inferior cerebellar artery, pontine perforating arteries, the base of the brain, dural sinuses, and the falx cerebri.

⚠ CAUTION

The use of opiate analgesia for managing poststroke headache should be avoided because the sedative effects may mask the clinical signs of neurological deterioration and may cause adverse effects such as respiratory depression and hypotension.

Sleep disorders

About 10 to 50% of stroke patients have sleep–wake disturbances, which negatively affect short- and long-term outcomes, length of hospitalization, and stroke recurrence risk. The spectrum of poststroke wakefulness disturbances includes hypersomnia, excessive daytime sleepiness, and fatigue. Poststroke hypersomnia can be found after subcortical (in particular caudate–putamen), thalamomesencephalic, upper pontine, medial pontomedullary, and even cortical strokes. Sleepiness can also be part of a top of the basilar syndrome. Other possible associations or precipitating factors include depression, anxiety, sleep-disordered breathing, drugs, poststroke pain, medical complications (urinary or respiratory infections, nocturia, dysphagia), and environmental factors such as noise and light. Poststroke sleep–wake disturbance management is a challenging therapeutic goal. There are no systematic studies or guidelines on the treatment of sleep disorders after stroke. Precipitating factors such as medical complications should be addressed first. Treatment of associated depression with antidepressants can improve poststroke sleeping problems and might be preferable for long-term management of poststroke insomnia. Nonpharmacological management should include avoidance of precipitating factors.

Poststroke insomnia incidence was reported to be 56.7%, with 18.1% reporting insomnia after their stroke, and 38.6% of patients reporting symptoms preceding stroke [21]. In view of the known consequences of impaired sleep, that is fatigue and attention and cognitive problems, insomnia likely impairs stroke recovery. Insomnia may be related directly to brain damage, particularly in the brainstem. Insomnia is defined by difficulty initiating or maintaining sleep, early awakenings, poor sleep quality, and daytime fatigue. Often poststroke insomnia is linked with stroke complications and not due to brain damage *per se*. Environmental factors (including noise, light, and intensive care unit monitoring) may play a role together with comorbidities such as cardiac failure, sleep disordered breathing, anxiety, depression, or pain. The recognition of poststroke insomnia occurs mainly on clinical grounds. Actigraphy may be used to document and quantify the reduction in sleep time and quality. Polysomnography is only rarely needed. Treatment of poststroke insomnia should include placement of patients in quiet rooms at night, protection from noise and light, light exposure and physical activity during the day, and, when unavoidable, temporary use of hypnotics that are relatively free of cognitive and muscle-relaxant effects, such as zolpidem. Benzodiazepines may provoke neuropsychological deficits and result in the re-emergence of motor symptoms. Sedative antidepressants may also improve poststroke insomnia.

Sleep-disordered breathing is highly prevalent in stroke patients and is both a risk factor and a consequence of stroke. Sleep-disordered breathing is common, particularly in elderly stroke male patients with diabetes, night-time stroke onset, and small vessel disease as cause of stroke. Sleep-disordered breathing improves after the acute phase of stroke, is associated with an increased poststroke mortality, and can be treated with continuous positive airway pressure (CPAP) in a small percentage of patients.

Sleep-disordered breathing, such as obstructive sleep apnea (OSA) and central sleep apnea, can occur as a consequence of stroke. Patients with stroke have an increased incidence of OSA compared with normal sex- and age-matched control subjects. The prevalence of OSA in patients with stroke is 50 to 70%. Primary risk factors for OSA include the male gender, over 40 years of age, overweight persons or recent weight gain, and persons with a large neck size or small chin/jaw. Cheyne–Stokes breathing is another poststroke complication characterized by cyclic fluctuations in breathing drive, hyperpneas alternating with apneas, or hypopneas in a gradual waxing and waning fashion. Stroke patients can present with obstructive sleep apnea, central sleep apnea, and Cheyne–Stokes breathing. Screening for sleep-disordered breathing may be warranted in all stroke patients who may potentially accept CPAP treatment. Sleep-disordered breathing can be accurately diagnosed by respiratory polygraphy, in which nasal airflow, respiratory movements, and capillary oxygen saturation are monitored. Polysomnography offers additional information, but is expensive and less commonly available. It should therefore be reserved for cases of diagnostic uncertainty. Oxygen saturation obtained from nocturnal pulse oximetry can be more easily used and is cheaper. Sleep-disordered breathing treatment in stroke patients represents a technical and logistical challenge. Treatment should always include prevention and therapy of secondary complications (respiratory infections, pain) and cautious use of sedative–hypnotic drugs, which negatively affect breathing during sleep. Patient positioning in the acute phase influences oxygen saturation as well.

Conclusion

Preventive measures to reduce medical and neurological complications in hospitalized patients with stroke may have beneficial effects on stroke outcomes and neurological recovery. Management of these complications represents an important aspect of the comprehensive care of the hospitalized patient with stroke. Admission of stroke patients to specialized stroke units can help minimize the impact of complications, wherein patients are closely monitored for early detection of these complications. Close observation for signs or symptoms of immobility (DVT, aspiration pneumonia, pressure sores and ulcerations, and falls) or infection (UTI, aspiration pneumonia) is necessary. Attention should be paid for possible nonbleeding complications of rt-PA, signs or symptoms of GI bleeding, or cardiac complications. Screening for delirium should be also considered and incorporated into the initial stroke assessment. Neurological deterioration should prompt assessment for cerebral edema, hemorrhagic transformation, or seizures.

Selected bibliography

1. Westendorp WF, Nederkoorn PJ, Vermeij JD, et al. Post-stroke infection: a systematic review and meta-analysis. *BMC Neurol* 2011; **11**: 110.
2. Diserens K, Moreira T, Hirt L, et al. Early mobilization out of bed after ischemic stroke reduces severe complications but not cerebral blood flow: a randomized controlled pilot trial. *Clin Rehabil* 2012; **26**: 451–9.
3. Adams HP Jr, del Zoppo G, Alberts MJ, et al. Guidelines for the early management of adults with ischemic stroke: a guideline from the American Heart Association/American Stroke Association Stroke Council, Clinical Cardiology Council, Cardiovascular Radiology and Intervention Council, and the Atherosclerotic Peripheral Vascular Disease and Quality of Care Outcomes in Research Interdisciplinary Working Groups: the American Academy of Neurology affirms the value of this guideline as an educational tool for neurologists. *Stroke* 2007; **38**: 1655–711.
4. Paciaroni M, Agnelli G, Venti M, et al. Efficacy and safety of anticoagulants in the prevention of venous thromboembolism in patients with acute cerebral hemorrhage: a meta-analysis of controlled studies. *J Thromb Haemost* 2011; **9**: 893–8.
5. Kamphuisen PW, Agnelli G. What is the optimal pharmacological prophylaxis for the prevention of deep-vein thrombosis and pulmonary embolism in patients with acute ischemic stroke? *Thromb Res* 2007; **119**: 265–74.
6. Sherman DG, Albers GW, Bladin C, et al. The efficacy and safety of enoxaparin versus unfractionated heparin for the prevention of venous thromboembolism after acute ischemic stroke (PREVAIL Study): an open-label randomized comparison. *Lancet* 2007; **369**: 1347–55.
7. Kase CS, Albers GW, Bladin C, et al. Neurological outcomes in patients with ischemic stroke receiving enoxaparin or heparin for venous thromboembolism prophylaxis: subanalysis of the Prevention of VTE after Acute Ischemic Stroke with LMWH (PREVAIL) study. *Stroke* 2009; **40**: 3532–40.
8. Nederkoorn PJ, Westendorp WF, Hooijenga IJ, et al. Preventive antibiotics in stroke study: rationale and protocol for a randomized trial. *Int J Stroke* 2011; **6**: 159–63.
9. Wip C, Napolitano L. Bundles to prevent ventilator-associated pneumonia: how valuable are they? *Curr Opin Infect Dis* 2009; **2**: 159–66.
10. Tutuarima JA, van der Meulen JH, de Haan RJ, et al. Risk factors for falls of hospitalized stroke patients. *Stroke* 1997; **28**: 297–301.
11. Schmid AA, Wells CK, Concato J, et al. Prevalence, predictors, and outcomes of post-stroke falls in acute hospital setting. *J Rehabil Res Dev* 2010; **47**: 553–62.
12. Cotter VT. Restraint free care in older adults with dementia. *Keio J Med* 2005; **54**: 80–4.
13. Kwok T, Mok F, Chien WT, et al. Does access to bed-chair pressure sensors reduce physical restraint use in the rehabilitative care setting? *J Clin Nurs* 2006; **15**: 581–7.
14. Dennis MS, Lewis SC, Warlow C. FOOD Trial Collaboration. Effect of timing and method of enteral tube feeding for dysphagic stroke patients (FOOD): a multicenter randomized controlled trial. *Lancet* 2005; **365**: 764–72.

15. Mc Manus J, Pathansali R, Hassan H, et al. The evaluation of delirium post-stroke. *Int J Geriatr Psychiatry* 2009; **24**: 1251–6.

16. Vahedi K, Hofmeijer J, Juettler E, et al. Early decompressive surgery in malignant infarction of the middle cerebral artery: a pooled analysis of three randomized controlled trials. *Lancet Neurol* 2007; **6**: 215–22.

17. Morgenstern LB, Hemphill JC 3rd, Anderson C, et al. Guidelines for the management of spontaneous intracerebral hemorrhage: a guideline for healthcare professionals from the American Heart Association/American Stroke Association. *Stroke* 2010; **41**: 2108–29.

18. Hacke W, Kaste M, Fieschi C, et al. Randomized double-blind placebo-controlled trial of thrombolytic therapy with intravenous alteplase in acute ischemic stroke (ECASS II). Second European-Australasian Acute Stroke Study Investigators. *Lancet* 1998; **352**: 1245–51.

19. Szaflarski JP, Rackley AY, Kleindorfer DO, et al. Incidence of seizures in the acute phase of stroke: a population-based study. *Epilepsia* 2008; **49**: 974–81.

20. Kumral E, Bogousslavsky J, Van Melle G, et al. Headache at stroke onset: the Lausanne Stroke Registry. *J Neurol Neurosurg Psychiatry* 1995; **58**: 490–2.

21. Leppävuori A, Pohjasvaara T, Vataja R, et al. Insomnia in ischemic stroke patients. *Cerebrovasc Dis* 2002; **14**: 90–7.

7

Poststroke Recovery

Samir R. Belagaje, MD[1] and Andrew J. Butler, PT, MBA, PhD, FAHA[2]

[1] Departments of Neurology and Rehabilitation Medicine, Emory University School of Medicine, Atlanta, Georgia
[2] B.F. Lewis School of Nursing and Health Professions, Georgia State University, Atlanta Georgia

Introduction

Stroke is a leading causes of disability world-wide. Stroke may produce ongoing functional disability due to persistent sensory, physical, language, cognitive, and emotional changes. About 50–70% of stroke survivors regain functional independence. However, for many people recovery is incomplete and the majority of patients do not return to pre-stroke levels of activity. Disability can range from severe deficits such as hemiplegia or aphasia to subtle cognitive slowing or sensory changes resulting in diminished quality of life. In the United States, the projected direct and indirect costs of stroke is over $1 trillion to the nation's health-care system burden over the next 50 years. The high prevalence, diminished quality of life, and economic costs of poststroke disabilities stress the importance that health-care practitioners involved in stroke care familiarize themselves with the mechanisms and interventions associated with the poststroke recovery process.

Unfortunately, knowledge of stroke recovery remains in its relative infancy and recovery remains a poorly defined concept. *Stroke recovery* could imply anything from the complete return of function and elimination of the cognitive, sensory, and motor impairments following brain injury, to very mild improvement in any of the associated motor or sickness behaviors. Depending on how successful recovery is defined, the proportion of patients classified as recovered in stroke outcome studies can vary markedly (see Evidence at a Glance). Consequently, stroke recovery could be best thought of as improvement across a profile of outcomes, beginning with biological and neurologic changes and appearing as improvement on performance and activity-based behavioral measures.

EVIDENCE AT A GLANCE

In their seminal paper, Duncan et al. compared patterns of recovery using different outcome measures and varying cut-off points to define successful recovery [1]. When recovery was defined at the disability level (i.e. Barthel Index greater than 90), the majority (57.3%) of stroke survivors in the study experienced a full recovery. Fewer individuals were considered to be fully recovered if measured by the degree of their impairment. If full recovery was defined as less than or equal to 1 on the National Institutes of Health Stroke Scale (NIHSS), 44.9% of study participants were fully recovered. Using a total Fugl–Meyer score greater than 90, 36.8% were fully recovered. Less than 25% of stroke survivors in the study were considered recovered if recovery was defined relative to reported prior function of physical activity. Utilizing the definition of recovery on the modified Rankin scale from ≤1 to ≤2 shifts the percentage of those deemed recovered from ≤25% to 53.8%.

Stroke, First Edition. Edited by Kevin M. Barrett and James F. Meschia.
© 2013 John Wiley & Sons, Ltd. Published 2013 by John Wiley & Sons, Ltd.

Table 7.1 Approaches to stroke rehabilitation

Strategy	Goals	Examples
Restoration (restitution)	1. Restore the function of damaged brain tissue 2. Retrain parts of the central nervous system to engage lost functions	1. Constraint-Induced therapy for upper extremity weakness 2. Speech therapy for dysphagia and aphasia
Compensation (substitution)	1. Adapt individual's behavior to the loss of function 2. Not changing the actual impairments	1. Training unaffected limb to perform activities such as feeding or writing 2. Use of gestures or writing to compensate for speech loss or dysarthria
Modification	1. Continue activities of daily living by changing the environment to accommodate 2. Use of assistive devices to navigate environments	1. Addition of ramps or shower stalls in the home 2. Use of prisms to minimize diplopia

The stroke recovery progression usually involves formal stroke rehabilitation. *Stroke rehabilitation* has been broadly defined as any aspect of stroke care (generally nonsurgical and nonpharmaceutical) that aims to reduce disability and promote participation in activities of daily living (ADLs). This chapter will depart from the traditional definition of stroke rehabilitation by including evidence to support the use of pharmaceuticals in the stroke rehabilitation process. The objective of stroke rehabilitation is to prevent deterioration of function as well as improve function while bringing about the highest possible level of independence, physically, psychologically, socially, and financially within the limits of the persistent stroke impairments. Stroke rehabilitation can be considered a process by which stroke survivors receive treatment and training to help them return to normal life by regaining and relearning skills of everyday living. Rehabilitation can be behaviorally beneficial for many stroke survivors, leading to greater independence in activities of daily living and improved functional capacity. Table 7.1 summarizes the approaches to rehabilitation.

Research is ongoing to understand various aspects of stroke recovery including: basic mechanisms underlying neuroplasticity and other mechanisms by which the brain repairs itself after a stroke, interventions to augment stroke recovery, and other factors which alter the stroke recovery trajectory. *Neuroplasticity* refers to the ability of the nervous system to change its structure, function, and connections in response to experience or the environment. Neuroplasticity may be used to describe changes at different levels of the nervous system, ranging from molecular events, to cellular events such as growth of new neurons (neurogenesis) and synapses (synaptogenesis), to behaviors.

★ TIPS AND TRICKS

When health-care practitioners think of stroke recovery, it is traditionally considered to be referrals to various types of rehabilitation therapy and a practice exclusively in the hands of rehabilitation specialists. Many believe that recovery from a stroke is possible only during a finite amount of time after the stroke onset (6–12 months) and after this initial period complete return of function may not be possible. Recent data have cast doubt on this assumption and the evidence suggests that stroke survivors can recover function beyond the 6-month time window. We believe that recovery begins immediately after a stroke occurs and advocate the rehabilitation process begin the moment a stroke patient encounters the health-care system, irrespective of acuity. Rehabilitation from a stroke is not the sole responsibility of therapists and physiatrists but should include all providers involved in stroke care.

This chapter will review and summarize the key concepts relating to poststroke recovery whose goal is the complete return of function and elimination of cognitive, sensory, and motor impairments. Traditional rehabilitation practices and therapeutic options have been reviewed in prior literature and our focus will be geared toward novel and emerging modalities available to enhance poststroke recovery. The structure of the chapter begins with an overview of the natural history of stroke recovery as well as the phases of stroke and their implications for rehabilitation. We then briefly review the mechanisms and current understanding of poststroke recovery principles. Finally, the chapter will conclude with a survey of emerging technology and interventions that may play a role in future poststroke recovery.

Natural history of stroke recovery

Observational studies have provided insight into the natural history of stroke and its subsequent outcomes. Consequently, certain clinical patterns of poststroke recovery have been characterized. It is generally believed that the first few weeks poststroke, the so-called acute–subacute period, is the time frame for the greatest rate of spontaneous recovery. In a cohort of 102 patients with ischemic middle cerebral artery (MCA) territory strokes, the amount of upper extremity functional recovery in the first 4 weeks was predictive of disability at 6 months [2].

General patterns are also seen with respect to the type of functional deficit with certain functional deficits demonstrating faster recovery rates. Proximal recovery usually occurs before distal recovery and lower extremity deficits have faster recovery in terms of disability measures when compared to upper extremity deficits.

EVIDENCE AT A GLANCE

Swallowing, facial movement, and gait tend to demonstrate better recovery. One hypothesis is that these deficits have bihemispheric representation in the cortex as part of their normal functional anatomy. Thus, after a stroke, when there is increased activation throughout the brain, tasks with bihemispheric representation are less affected and show clinical improvement. Similarly, compared to the dominant hand, the nondominant hand is normally bilaterally organized and remains that way after a stroke. Eloquent cortical functions such as language, dominant hand movement, and spatial attention are more lateralized in function and recover more slowly.

Although great strides in recovery are seen initially, most stroke survivors who do not achieve early and complete spontaneous recovery reach a plateau phase without additional significant spontaneous improvement. In the Copenhagen Stroke Study, a cohort study of over 1100 hospitalized acute stroke patients found maximum arm motor function within 9 weeks poststroke in 95% of patients. Among those with lower extremity paresis recovery of walking function occurred in 95% of the patients within the first 11 weeks after stroke. The time and the degree of recovery were associated with the degree of functional walking impairment and the severity of lower extremity paresis. Similar findings have been observed in patients with aphasia or neglect, with recovery plateaus occurring at approximately 6 weeks and 3 months, respectively. Prediction of recovery in the upper extremity is dependent on baseline impairment. The Fugl–Meyer score at the time of initial impairment of upper extremity was found to be a good predictor of motor recovery in nonsevere hemiparesis. However, it is less predictive in patients with more severe deficits. A summary of key features and detailed items of the upper-extremity subscale of the Fugl–Meyer motor assessment (UE-FM) is provided in Table 7.2.

The period of greatest recovery in the first 3 months can be augmented by therapy. In the seminal meta-analysis of 36 clinical trials examining

Table 7.2 Summary of key features and detailed items of the upper-extremity subscale of the Fugl–Meyer motor assessment (UE-FM)

Parameter	UE-FM
Number of Items	33
Scale	Ordinal 3-point
Score range	0–66
Time required to administer (min)	12–15
Measure	Impairment
	1. Shoulder retraction
	2. Shoulder elevation
	3. Shoulder abduction
	4. Shoulder abduction to 90°
	5. Shoulder adduction/internal rotation
	6. Shoulder external rotation
	7. Shoulder flexion 0–90°
	8. Shoulder flexion 90–180°
	9. Elbow flexion
	10. Elbow extension
	11. Forearm supination
	12. Forearm pronation
	13. Forearm supination/pronation (elbow at 0°)
	14. Forearm supination/pronation (elbow at 90°)
	15. Hand to lumbar spine
	16. Wrist flexion/extension (elbow at 0°)
	17. Wrist flexion/extension (elbow at 90°)
	18. Wrist extension against resistance (elbow at 90°)
	19. Wrist extension against resistance (elbow at 90°)
	20. Wrist circumduction
	21. Finger flexion
	22. Finger extension
	23. Extension of MCP joints, flexion of PIP or DIP joints
	24. Grasp: adduct thumb
	25. Grasp: oppose thumb
	26. Grasp cylinder
	27. Grasp tennis ball
	28. Finger-to-nose speed
	29. Finger-to-nose tremor
	30. Finger-to-nose dysmetria
	31. Finger flexion reflex
	32. Biceps reflex
	33. Triceps reflex

UE-FM, upper extremity Fugl–Meyer assessment; MCP, metacarpophalangeal; PIP, proximal interphalangeal; DIP, distal interphalangeal.
Reprinted by permission from Lin JH, MJ Hsu, et al. (2009). *Phys Ther* **89**(8): 840–50.

the effectiveness of stroke rehabilitation, people receiving poststroke rehabilitation were shown to have higher levels of function than 65% of those stroke survivors who did not receive rehabilitation [3]. This important finding was seen across several measures, including ambulation, self-care ability, communication, and independence. Recognizing that earlier recovery offers a better prognosis and rehabilitation also improves outcomes, additional studies are needed to further understand the optimal timing and amount of rehabilitation with respect to frequency and intensity. Paolucci et al. examined differences in outcomes for patients for whom therapy was initiated 20 days apart and found a strong inverse relationship between the start date and functional outcome, albeit with wide confidence intervals [4]. In other words, those who initiated therapy soon after stroke ictus exhibited significantly higher effectiveness of treatment than did the medium or late-initiating groups. Treatment initiated within the first 20 days was associated with a significantly high probability of excellent therapeutic response (odds ratio (OR)=6.11; 95% CI, 2.03 to 18.36), and beginning at 20 or 40 days was associated with a poor response (OR=5.18; 95% CI, 1.07 to 25.00) [4].

Phases of stroke: implications for rehabilitation

When characterizing the various time periods after stroke, there is a discrepancy between the neurology and the rehabilitation medical communities about the length of time apportioned to each phase. These differences arise as a consequence of the nature of the roles and interventions the various medical specialties use. These differences are seen in the literature and may serve as a potential source of confusion when engaging in discussion concerning stroke rehabilitation across the various disciplines. For the purposes of clarity and consistency, the following terms will be employed in this chapter to define phase of stroke onset and recovery as has been generally accepted in the literature (Table 7.3).

Hyperacute: <24 hours after stroke onset
Acute: 24 hours to 4 weeks after stroke onset
Subacute: 1 month to 3 months after stroke onset
Chronic: >3 months after stroke onset.

Hyperacute phase (<24 hours after stroke onset)

In the hyperacute phase of stroke, patients may be medically unstable and rehabilitation is not

Table 7.3 Summary of key recommendations during stroke recovery

Phase	Key recommendations	Key points
Hyperacute	Early mobilization is safe Early impairments and disability can accurately predict recovery Neuroimaging can assist with prognosis	Early mobilization appears to be safe and beneficial but not completely proven
Acute	Screen for early signs of depression and treat aggressively Avoid sedative medications when possible	Depression can worsen outcomes and occurs at any phase There may be a role for neurostimulation to improve arousal and concentration but not proven yet
Subacute	Constraint-induced therapy should be considered for appropriate individuals with upper extremity hemiparesis Medications should be considered as an adjunct to standard therapy as well as to treat depression	While constraint-induced therapy has been shown beneficial in subacute and chronic stages, the same effect has not been demonstrated in earlier phases
Chronic	Spasticity can worsen outcomes and can be addressed with medications	This phase is when a lot of stroke survivors hit a plateau in their recovery; however, it is possible that they continue to make improvements and advance with novel therapies and continued work

typically a major consideration. It is often given secondary importance to considerations regarding acute thrombolytic and reperfusion strategies. In the hyperacute phase of stroke, patients and families often inquire about prognosis for deficits that remain despite acute stroke interventions. Recent data suggest that prognosis can be made for some motor deficits using simple bedside tests. The Early Prediction of Functional Outcome after Stroke (EPOS) study found that recovery of upper extremity function at 6 months could be accurately predicted if voluntary finger extension and shoulder abduction were present at 48 hours poststroke [5]. In fact, if these movements were present, the probability of a good outcome was 98% and if finger extension was not present within 48 hours, the probability of a good outcome was 25%. If the movements did not improve by day 9 poststroke the likelihood of complete upper extremity recovery decreased to 14% [5].

🔬 SCIENCE REVISITED

In a study involving patients with first ischemic stroke causing upper extremity weakness, the change in Fugl–Meyer (FM) score could be ascertained using initial FM scores in combination with a functional MRI recovery measure [6]. In patients with less severe deficits, 96% of the total sum of squares of the change in FM was explained by the initial FM score. However, in patients with more severe deficits, the initial FM score only explained 16% of change in FM scores. In patients with severe deficit, adding fMRI recovery measure increased predictive explanation from 16% to 47% of the total sum of squares of change in FM; although the increase was not statistically significant.

Prediction of motor recovery in the hyperacute phase can also be assisted by utilizing routine neuroimaging. A small case series showed that brain magnetic resonance imaging (MRI) could be useful in predicting recovery early after a stroke. In 20 subjects with stroke, apparent diffusion coefficient (ADC) maps were calculated from diffusion-weighted images (DWI) acquired <6 hours, 12 hours, 24 hours, and 7 days after stroke. Signal intensity

values were calculated within three regions of interest in the descending corticospinal tract between the upper midbrain and cervicomedullary junction. These values were then correlated with NIHSS motor scores 3 months after stroke. Poor recovery defined as NIHSS scores >2 for both the arm and leg was associated with a decrease in ADC signal in the ipsilesional cerebral peduncle that peaked 7 days after stroke with high positive and negative predictive values [7]. ADC maps can be readily constructed from DWI included in a routine clinical series, and a decrease in signal can be reliably identified within 7 days of stroke. Advanced neuroimaging modalities and new technologies can improve prediction but have not been incorporated into routine clinical practice and are considered investigational. Additional examples will be discussed in more detail later in the chapter.

Consensus is lacking as to when to start rehabilitation after stroke. The American Heart Association/American Stroke Association stroke care guidelines state that "...early mobilization is favored..," but specific recommendations for early mobilization are not provided. It is often assumed that stroke patients who receive thrombolytic therapy should not be mobilized for at least 24 hours to minimize tissue plasminogen activator (tPA) complications. For example, post-thrombolytic patients have strict blood pressure criteria to minimize risk of hemorrhage development. Therefore, clinicians are wary to increase physical activity in patients that may lead to an elevation in blood pressure. Patients treated with endovascular arterial reperfusion often are confined to bedrest to minimize the risk of complications related to femoral access.

Recent clinical trials have demonstrated that early mobilization is beneficial for functional recovery in carefully selected patients with stroke. In the A Very Early Rehabilitation Trial (AVERT), a multicenter, phase II, randomized trial, hospitalized patients were randomized to receive customary therapy or very early mobilization (VEM). Those assigned to VEM were mobilized as soon as practical after randomization with the goal of within 24 hours following stroke onset. Furthermore, the VEM group received additional assistance, with the aim of being upright and out of bed at least twice per day – double the "mobilization dose" compared to those in the standard care (SC) arm. A trained nurse and physiotherapy team delivered the intervention for the first

14 days after stroke or until discharge from the acute stroke unit. The number of study participants receiving IV tPA was estimated to be about 10%. For the safety outcome there was no significant difference in the number of deaths between groups (SC, 3/33 (9%); VEM, 8/38 (21%); $P=0.20$). The number of falls, early neurologic deterioration, and patient fatigue were not significantly different between groups. Subsequent analyses have demonstrated that exposure to very early and intensive mobilization led to a significantly faster return to walking than did standard stroke care ($P=0.032$; median 3.5 vs. 7.0 days) [8]. VEM was independently associated with good functional outcome on the Barthel Index at 3 months ($P=0.008$) [8].

Secondary analyses have shown the value of early mobilization in terms of cost–benefit analyses and feasibility and were sustainable at 1 year. Comparable findings were found in the smaller Very Early Rehabilitation or Intensive Telemetry after Stroke (VERITAS) study. A larger AVERT Phase III trial involving multiple centers is currently underway.

The preliminary results from AVERT demonstrated that mobilization within 24 hours following stroke onset is safe and may potentially improve clinical outcomes. However, caution must be taken with respect to the intensity and amount of therapy. Based on the results of the Very Early Constraint Induced Movement Therapy (VECTORS) trial, it appears that more therapy does not always equate with better outcomes [9]. The details of this trial and its implications will be discussed in the acute rehabilitation section of the chapter.

The hyperacute period of stroke recovery may be an opportunity to introduce pharmacological agents to promote recovery. Many medications are more appropriate in the intensive care unit setting where stimulants are often used to increase alertness and attention. Attention modulates neural signals and is essential for learning and memory. In stroke patients brain lesions that subserve attention networks may have been interrupted. A small clinical trial explored the use of neurostimulants to decrease the length of stay in the intensive care unit for patients with traumatic brain injury. To date, strong evidence for use of neurostimulants in hyperacute stroke care does not exist. However, the use of neurostimulants to influence attention in the hyperacute phase warrants further investigation.

CAUTION

Certain pharmacological interventions may slow or impair poststroke recovery when administered in the hyperacute phase. In the acute–hyperacute phase, benzodiazepines and other hypnotic-sedative medications are commonly used to treat insomnia and agitation. Clinical trials have found that benzodiazepines can hinder neuroplasticity. The exact mechanism has not been clearly established, but gamma-aminobutryic acid (GABA) transmission may play a critical role through inhibition of synaptogenesis and brain circuitry. The use of hypnotics, anxiolytics, and sedative medications in the acute–hyperacute phase should be avoided when possible.

The hyperacute period is also the time period to initiate many of the practical, standards-of-care to reduce disability and promote participation in activities of daily living. A standard measure used by The Joint Commission (TJC) for primary stroke center certification is the evaluation of swallowing function before administering parenteral (PO) intake and food. A prompt evaluation of swallowing function allows a speech therapist to begin assessing with more formal testing, such as barium swallow, and to initiate dysphagia therapy if necessary. Assessment of swallowing function and implementation of dietary modification can reduce the incidence of aspiration pneumonia. Such infections have been shown to adversely impact stroke recovery and poststroke outcomes. In a similar fashion, it is not unreasonable to begin consultations with physical and occupational therapy.

Emerging evidence suggests that early mobilization and rehabilitation is safe and effective in the hyperacute period following stroke. Neuroimaging and functional impairment such as voluntary finger extension and shoulder abduction can be useful in predicting eventual recovery. Additional studies are needed before pharmacologic strategies to promote recovery in the hyperacute stroke phase can be recommended.

Acute phase (24 hours to 4 weeks after stroke onset)

In the acute phase of stroke recovery the majority of medical issues have stabilized and rehabilitation is typically performed in an in-patient facility. During this phase, a complete evaluation of the stroke etiology is undertaken and stroke risk factors are addressed. During the acute phase, traditional rehabilitation plays a prominent role in promoting successful recovery. Evidence suggests new intervention strategies may serve an even larger role in recovery following stroke than has been typically utilized.

Mood disorders such as depression are increasingly being recognized as common sequelae of stroke recovery in the acute phase. The prevalence of clinically diagnosed poststroke depression ranges from 20 to 40% and is likely underdiagnosed. Recovery is often hindered in patients whose depression is under- or untreated. Symptoms of depression such as fatigue, reduced motivation, and loss of confidence can negatively impact the benefits of rehabilitation in the acute phase. Depression and anxiety are characterized by attention and concentration difficulties. Studies have shown that poststroke depression can cause higher rates of mortality and morbidity. Treatment of depression leads to improved functional recovery after stroke through restored balance of central neurotransmitters, improved motivation to work with rehabilitation therapists, and better adherence to medications.

Selective serotonin receptor inhibitors (SSRIs) have been the most-studied agents for treatment of poststroke depression. Citalopram is superior to placebo in treating poststroke depression as measured by the Hamilton Depression scale. Positive results with regard to improved quality of life after administration of sertraline in patients with poststroke depression has been reported. In contrast, conflicting data are seen in multiple trials when fluoxetine was used to treat poststroke depression. Evidence supports the efficacy of tricyclic antidepressants for treatment of poststroke depression. Nortriptyline 100 mg/day was superior to fluoxetine or placebo in one study and imipramine had demonstrated benefit in another study. Single-case studies have reported the efficacy of reboxetine, a norepinephrine reuptake inhibitor, as well as methylphenidate.

⚓ CAUTION

Tricyclic antidepressants have extensive side-effect profiles and should not be considered first-line treatment for poststroke depression. They should be used with caution, particularly in the elderly and patients with a history of cardiac conduction abnormalities.

Cognitive impairments are a common consequence of stroke in the acute phase. Cognitive difficulties have been found to be present in a significant proportion of stroke patients. Attention skills, including divided attention, sustained attention, selective attention, and speed of information processing, are commonly impaired. Neurostimulants are commonly used during the acute stroke recovery period in an attempt to increase arousal, alertness, and attention in patients. Examples of neurostimulants that have been studied in the poststroke population include methylphenidate, bromocriptine, amantadine, carbidopa/levodopa, and Provigil. Unfortunately, while small studies have suggested improvement, larger studies have not confirmed the benefit.

EVIDENCE AT A GLANCE

Analysis of data from the Post-Stroke Rehabilitation Outcomes Project (PSROP) showed that patients treated with neurostimulant medications did not exhibit significant changes in length of stay, motor recovery, cognitive recovery, or discharge destination when compared to patients who did not receive neurostimulants. The database included >1200 poststroke rehabilitation patients (mean age = 66 years, 52% male, 60% Caucasian, and 23% Black) who were treated between 2001 and 2003 in seven inpatient rehabilitation facilities [10]. Limitations include the retrospective study design and the use of neurostimulants in a minority (20%) of patients.

Certain medications used in the acute period have been shown to impede poststroke recovery. The prevalence of poststroke seizures is about 10%. Inadequate treatment of seizures following stroke in the hyperacute–acute phase of recovery can lengthen length of hospital stay and delay rehabilitation. Antiepileptic drugs such as phenytoin, phenobarbital, and diazepam have been shown to hinder neuroplastic synaptic formation in animal models by virtue of their target neurotransmitters. Newer generation AEDs should be considered when treatment is necessary to avoid detrimental effects on poststroke recovery.

Antihistamines, such as H2-blockers, are commonly prescribed during stroke hospitalizations to prevent gastric reflux and to counter potential gastrointestinal side-effects of antithrombotic medications such as aspirin. Since antithrombotics are an evidence-based intervention for secondary stroke prevention, the use of H2 blockers is widespread. Antihistamines can cause sedation in elderly patients and compromise attention vital for effective performance of motor and cognitive tasks such as learning. As discussed previously, sedation can hinder active participation in rehabilitation and response to rehabilitation therapy. There is evidence to suggest that these medications can impede plasticity through inhibition of long-term potentiation.

★ TIPS AND TRICKS

One possible solution to reduce sedative effects is the use of proton pump inhibitors as an alternative to the antihistamines as they have the desirable antiacid properties without the untoward side-effects of sedation and cognitive impairment, which could impede poststroke recovery.

Subacute phase (1 month to 3 months after stroke onset)

During the subacute rehabilitation phase of stroke recovery patients are commonly stable and have been discharged from the hospital. For those patients with mild motor deficits, they will have likely returned home and continue to receive therapy as an out-patient. For those survivors with more severe deficits, they may be in an acute rehabilitation facility or a skilled nursing facility. The focus in this phase of poststroke recovery is to improve function. Traditionally, the subacute phase has been primarily when patients spend the bulk of their time receiving therapy to reduce disability and promote participation in activities of daily living (ADL). Families are taught to assist with transfers and continue therapy of the stroke survivor.

In the past decade, a class of high-intensity, focused interventions has emerged that have been initiated in the subacute phase of stroke recovery. Many of these high-intensity interventions are based upon the paradigm of constraint-induced therapy (CIT). CIT is based on forced-use therapy and the theory of learned nonuse where patients become accustomed to not using their impaired limb and develop compensatory strategies such as using the nonparetic limb for ADLs. The goal of CIT is to restore function of the more impaired limb and damaged brain tissue by forcing patients to use their paretic limb as their nonparetic limb is "constrained" by a mitt or a sling.

EVIDENCE AT A GLANCE

In the Extremity Constraint Induced Therapy (EXCITE) trial, a randomized, single-blind, multicenter clinical trial, patients with residual upper extremity hemiparesis 3–9 months poststroke were randomized to CIT or standard therapy. From baseline to 12 months, the group receiving constraint-induced therapy showed greater improvements as measured by the Wolf Motor Function Test as well as the Motor Activity Log (MAL) Amount of Use (52% reduction in mean time vs. 26% reduction; $P < 0.001$) and in the MAL Amount of Use, between-group difference, 0.43 (95% CI, 0.05–0.80; $P < 0.001$). The CIT group achieved a decrease of 19.5 as measured by the Stroke Impact Scale in self-perceived hand function difficulty vs. a decrease of 10.1 for the control group ($P = 0.05$) [11].

Less intensive forms of CIT referred to as modified constraint-induced therapy (mCIT) has been shown to be of benefit for functional recovery. mCIT consists of restraint of the unaffected arm and hand 5 days/week × 5 hours during times of frequent use. The mCIT studies have been performed in stroke survivors in the subacute as well as the chronic phase of recovery. Feasibility and improvement in arm function as measured by Fugl–Meyer, Action Research Arm Test (ARAT), and motor activity log compared to traditional therapy has been established for mCIT. These studies are limited by small sample size and lack of randomization in the study design. mCIT may achieve greater adherence to treatment by reducing the time of constraint compared to traditional CIT. To date, direct comparison of mCIT and CIT protocols have not been performed.

Given the established benefits of CIT one may ask why it should not be initiated earlier in the course of poststroke recovery. Results from the Very Early Constraint Induced Movement during Stroke Rehabilitation (VECTORS) trial did not find incremental benefit with earlier intervention. VECTORS was a single-blind, phase II, randomized trial comparing traditional upper extremity therapy with dose-matched and high-intensity CIT protocols administered over the course of 2 weeks. Patients were randomized on average 9.65 ± 4.5 days after stroke onset. While both groups improved with time as measured by the ARAT score, the high-intensity CIT group had significantly less improvement at day 90. There were no significant differences between the dose-matched CIT and control groups at day 90 [9]. A complete understanding of the results of the VECTORS trial has not been reached. However, animal models have also demonstrated enlargement in areas of ischemia when constraint therapy is applied early after a stroke that correlates with poor functional outcomes. Based on these results, one could argue that CIT should be initiated in the subacute phase although more data are needed before any definite conclusions about early application of intense therapy such as CIT can be fully made.

The subacute period following stroke can provide an opportunity for pharmacological interventions to promote stroke recovery. For instance, memantine can serve as an adjunct for aphasia rehabilitation. While the mechanism remains unclear, it is hypothesized that its antiglutamate properties reduce glutamate-induced neurotoxicity seen in stroke. In a small study of 20 patients in the subacute phase, improvement in language function when combined with speech therapy as measured by the Western Aphasia Battery–Aphasia Quotient and the Communicative Activity Log was found when combined with speech therapy [12]. Likewise, the use of piracetam has been shown to be effective for the treatment of aphasia in a single randomized controlled trial; however, because the medication is not approved by the Food and Drug Administration (FDA), routine clinical use of this medication in the United States is inapplicable. The exact mechanism is unclear but its cholinergic properties and increase activation of excitatory neurotransmitters have been postulated as reasons for its role in improving aphasia.

Chronic phase (>3 months after stroke onset)

In the chronic phase of rehabilitation a constancy in the state of recovery may emerge. Many patients have completed or will be finishing their prescribed stroke out-patient therapy. It was once believed that patients who entered the plateau phase did not have the capacity for further improvement, thus any residual functional deficits were permanent. However, research in the past decade has shown this perception to be a misconception. There is mounting evidence that patients can continue to show functional improvement beyond the 3-month poststroke time period.

Spasticity often arises during the chronic phase of poststroke recovery. Spasticity is best defined as a motor disorder characterized by a velocity-dependent increase in tonic stretch reflexes with exaggerated tendon jerks, resulting from hyperexcitability of the stretch reflex. Untreated spasticity worsens stroke outcomes and has a negative impact on functional recovery. The optimal timing of treatment – before or in conjunction with the initiation of physical therapy – has yet to established.

Patients without spasticity have shown significantly better motor and activity scores when compared to those with spasticity. Patients with spasticity were more likely to receive institutional care and had significantly lower Barthel Index (BI) scores at 12 months ($P <0.0001$) [13]. Similarly, in another study, the proportion of patients with dependence in everyday activities according to modified Rankin scores (mRS) scores and BI was greater for patients with spasticity than for patients with no spasticity. From these studies, it is clear that spasticity does affect functional outcomes in the chronic phase and therefore strategies to manage spasticity are relevant to achievement of poststroke rehabilitation goals.

While treatment of spasticity has historically included oral medications such as baclofen, nerve blocks, and serial casting, these treatments are limited because of patient tolerability and side-effects. As an alternative, two additional options have gained widespread acceptance in managing spasticity in chronic stroke patients: intrathecal baclofen and botulinum toxin. When baclofen is administered intrathecally, muscle-relaxing properties have been achieved at significantly lower doses than the oral route, thereby limiting the systemic side-effects. Studies of intrathecal baclofen have demonstrated improved mobility, activities of daily living, and quality of life in spastic poststroke patients. In their recent approval of botulinum toxin for poststroke spasticity, the FDA cited three studies that showed improvement in upper limb musculature tone as measured by the modified Ashworth scale and physician global assessment of treatment response. In these studies, patients were at least 6 weeks poststroke (although one of the studies used 6 months poststroke as inclusion criteria) with modified Ashworth scale of 2–3 in upper extremity muscles of interest. Botulinum toxin was administered into muscles of interest in the hand, wrist, and upper arm and patients were followed for at least 10 weeks. Compared to placebo, there was a median reduction in the Ashworth scale from 0.5 to 2 depending on the joint. The results demonstrate that botulinum toxin improved outcome in patients at least 6 weeks poststroke.

Mechanisms of stroke recovery

In the past two decades, research has helped uncover some of the mechanisms of stroke recovery. It has become evident that multiple pathways and mechanisms are involved in poststroke recovery. Normal functions such as motor activity, attention, and language are mediated by multiple neuronal pathways distributed widely throughout the brain in a complex network. When an injury such as a stroke occurs to the brain, there is increased activation in the uninjured or remaining nodes to preserve function. Injuries from stroke also cause diaschisis which is the phenomenon of reduced blood flow and metabolism in uninjured brain areas which are reciprocally connected to the ischemic areas. Recovery has been associated with resolution of the diaschisis; in other words, a normalization of blood flow to these areas.

Initially following a stroke, there is reduced activation in directly injured cortical areas. This is accompanied by a change in the localization of certain tasks such as movement or function. Specifically, certain functions such as language or unilateral movement of a limb are lateralized to a particular hemisphere. For instance, traditional neuroscience principles place functions such as right-side movement and language in the left (dominant) hemisphere. After a stroke, there appears to be decreased lateralization of such functions and consequently multiple areas of homologous function within the network are activated.

As recovery occurs through the acute and subacute period, the neural networks, which had been disrupted by the stroke, reconnect in areas adjacent to the area of stroke. For example, functional neuroimaging techniques shows that as use of the hand improves, cortical representation that once subserved the hand relocate toward the cortical face area. Studies have shown that the degree of recovery is associated with the amount of activation to the peri-infarcted areas. Generally speaking, the more widely distributed brain activation in the neural network following a stroke, the less functional recovery is noted.

These changes in the neural network, which as described earlier are a group of neurons working together to perform a similar function, are the basis of neuroplasticity – the main process through which poststroke recovery occurs. Neuroplasticity may also be conceptualized as a remapping or rewiring of injured neural networks. Neuroplasticity is driven by certain principles confirmed by multiple animal studies. These principles can guide development and design of therapeutic interventions for recovery. Animal studies have shown that in order to promote plasticity, interventions must be task-specific and goal-directed rather than general and nonspecific movements. Furthermore, the goal-directed tasks must be challenging and interesting enough to maintain attention. Finally, the task should allow for multiple attempts or repetition.

Emerging technology

In this section, we will discuss the investigational strategies with the potential to improve prognostic estimates, further enhance poststroke recovery, and improve the rehabilitation process.

Predicting motor recovery of the upper limb after stroke rehabilitation with emerging technology

There are multiple factors affecting stroke recovery that often makes prognosticating outcome difficult. Nevertheless, clinicians often are asked to predict recovery following a stroke. In addition, the finite resources in a cost-containing health-care environment put a premium on allocating resources appropriately. Ensuring rehabilitation resources are directed towards patients with the most potential for recovery will be a guiding principle in future health care. To aid in this goal, clinicians will likely need to incorporate emerging and novel technology to assist with prognosis.

fMRI to predict stroke recovery

Brain-mapping techniques have proven to be vital in understanding the molecular, cellular, and functional mechanisms of recovery after stroke. Brain-mapping techniques, such as fMRI, also have the potential to predict recovery from stroke. It was discovered in the early 1990s that water in blood has different MRI imaging characteristics; a change in blood oxygenation leads to change in blood oxygenation-level dependent (BOLD) signal on MRI. When a region of brain tissue is active it requires more oxygenated blood and, subsequently, when it is less active oxygenated blood flow will decrease in that area. Because fMRI can detect this BOLD signal, it can measure activated brain areas for various tasks.

EVIDENCE AT A GLANCE

In a study of the prognostic utility of fMRI, chronic-phase stroke subjects underwent a baseline fMRI and then a repeat assessment following 6 weeks of therapy for upper arm rehabilitation. In addition to the imaging, patients underwent clinical assessments including the upper extremity Fugl–Myer. Using a multiple linear regression model, the degree of baseline motor cortex activation on fMRI was inversely associated with larger clinical gains [14]; in other words, the lower brain activation, the greater behavioral gains are seen. It was hypothesized that the lower cortical activation at baseline represents an under-use of surviving cortical tissue that will be used be used for repairing the brain after stroke. Based on the results of this study and those previously described, both lower activation as well as focused cortical activation are correlated with improved functional recovery following stroke.

Stroke recovery is correlated with certain fMRI activation patterns in the brain. These imaging patterns may be useful surrogates to determine if a therapeutic intervention is beneficial. For instance,

in a study of seven chronic hemiparetic patients who had fMRI while performing a hand flexion–extension movement before and after a 2-week home-based CIT program, improvement in hand function as measured by grip strength and the Jebsen–Taylor hand test after therapy varied between patients. However, in those patients with improved hand function, focused fMRI signal were shown in the contralateral premotor cortex and secondary somatosensory cortex as well as the areas in the bilateral cerebellar hemisphere [15].

The role of DTI in evaluation of stroke recovery

Another imaging technique with potential utility for assessing stroke recovery is diffusion tensor imaging (DTI), a type of sequence that can be done with MRI. Diffusion tensor imaging (DTI) allows for the visualization and quantitative examination of fiber tracts and their integrity via fractional anisotropy measures in vivo so that the topographic relation of lesion location and corticospinal fibers can be evaluated and fiber degeneration can be revealed.

In recent years, data have emerged putting the focus on neuroanatomy and the integrity of various structures. For instance, in patients with motor deficits, the integrity of motor cortex and corticospinal tracts are very important. In a seminal study, patients in the chronic phase with motor evoked potentials (MEPs) had the potential to continue to make meaningful strides in their recovery process [16]. Patients without MEPs as elicited by transcranial magnetic stimulation (TMS), integrity of the corticospinal tract as measured by DTI was predictive of recovery [16]. It was notable in this study that subjects were in the chronic phase of stroke.

EVIDENCE AT A GLANCE

The use of DTI for predicting motor recovery may provide more useful information than fMRI following supratentorial brain injury. In a study involving patients 3 to 9 months after stroke, upper extremity function was measured with Wolf Motor Function Test (WMFT) and the Fugl–Meyer (FM) score. Structural integrity of the posterior limb of the internal capsule (PLIC) was assessed by examining the fractional anisotropy (FA) asymmetry with DTI. Laterality index of motor cortical areas was measured as the BOLD response with fMRI in each patient during a finger pinch task. Strong relationships between clinical outcome measures and FA asymmetry (FM score ($R^2 = 0.655$, $P = 0.001$) and WMFT asymmetry score ($R^2 = 0.651$, $P < 0.002$)) were found, but relationships with fMRI measures were weaker. Based on their findings, the authors concluded that clinical motor function is more closely related to the white matter integrity of the internal capsule than to BOLD response of motor areas [17].

Emerging treatments and technology for stroke rehabilitation

Noninvasive brain stimulation

Transcranial magnetic stimulation
Noninvasive brain stimulation is an emerging adjunctive tool for both assessing brain changes following stroke and has the potential as a therapeutic modality to enhance stroke rehabilitation. Transcranial magnetic stimulation (TMS) utilizes magnetic pulses to generate electrical fields in the brain to excite cortical neurons. TMS may be applied over the motor cortex, generating motor evoked potentials (MEPs) in peripheral muscles. In addition to enhancing the understanding of neurophysiology in noninjured brains, the TMS can be used for prognostic and therapeutic interventions in stroke survivors.

Single-pulse TMS to predict stroke recovery
In the stroke literature, MEPs generated by TMS have been correlated with function and theorized to predict recovery. Recent literature demonstrates that the detection of MEPs in peripheral muscles upon stimulation of the injured cerebral cortex is a sign of favorable prognosis in subjects with stroke. It has been speculated that functional potential in chronic stroke patients may depend on corticospinal tract integrity from the initial, primary cortical representation of the clinically lesioned muscle, and has been shown in the DTI study described above. The integrity of the corticospinal tract is represented by the presence of MEPs.

Repetitive transcranial magnetic stimulation
In addition to being used for diagnostic purposes, another use of TMS may be for direct treatment purposes. Stroke alters the balance between excitation and inhibition between the hemispheres, which suggests that down-regulation of the unaffected primary motor cortex (M1) may facilitate motor recovery following stroke. Repetitive stimulation of a brain region within a short period of time (seconds) can increase or decrease the excitability of the neurons within that region depending on the intensity of stimulation, coil orientation, and frequency. This technique is referred to as repetitive TMS (rTMS). The ability of rTMS to modulate motor cortical excitability in a frequency-dependent manner has been utilized in studies investigating stimulation of either the affected or unaffected hemispheres of stroke patients. In several studies, the cortical plasticity changes have shown to last several weeks. Although data are preliminary, TMS may serve as a therapeutic option.

In a series of clinical trials, when compared to sham stimulation, rTMS has been shown to improve hand movement in stroke survivors. Low-frequency rTMS decreases cortical excitability and has been applied to the unaffected motor cortex to decrease hyperexcitability in chronic stroke patients. A single session of 1 Hz rTMS decreased cortical excitability and transcortical inhibition, and led to a short-lasting increase in pinch acceleration of the paretic hand, while no change was seen following sham stimulation. Other studies have investigated multiple treatment sessions in chronic stroke patients but only a few that have been applied to those in the acute stroke phase. The results of published studies to date show that rTMS gives a 10–30% improvement over sham stimulation across measures, from simple reaction times to timed behavioral tests. These studies suggest that decreasing inhibition in the affected M1, and perhaps other motor related areas such as the dorsal premotor cortex, can unmask pre-existing, functionally latent neural connections around the lesion and contribute to cortical reorganization. In a trial of 26 chronic stroke survivors, poststroke dysphagia improved for up to 2 months after multiple, daily 3 Hz excitatory rTMS to the lesioned hemisphere [18].

In addition to motor recovery, rTMS has been shown to have potential applications for treatment in neglect and aphasia. The FDA has recently approved certain protocols of rTMS as a treatment of refractory depression. However, to date there are no approved uses of rTMS for poststroke upper or lower limb recovery. The main risks associated with this procedure include head pain and a theoretical risk of seizures.

Transcranial direct current stimulation

Direct electrical current can stimulate cortical neurons, similar to TMS. This technique, known as transcranial direct current stimulation (tDCS), involves production of constant, low-amplitude, direct current through electrodes. When these electrodes are placed in the region of interest, the current induces intracerebral current flow. Whereas TMS uses a magnetic field to induce electric current flow, the electric current in tDCS is directly applied to the scalp overlying the brain region of interest. It is similar to TMS in that the result of the current induces changes in the neuronal excitability that may persist after the stimulation has been discontinued, likely through long-term potentiation mechanisms. With tDCS, neuronal excitability can be increased with anodal stimulation or decreased with cathodal stimulation.

Based on the rationale described above, tDCS has been studied in stroke survivors as a potential therapy adjunct to enhance neuroplastic changes essential for recovery. After reaching a training plateau on the Jebsen–Taylor Hand Function Test (JTT) a group of chronic stroke survivors received a single session of anodal tDCS in a double-blind protocol to motor regions of the affected cerebral hemisphere while continuing to perform the JTT. The investigators concluded that stimulation led to improvements in pinch force, Jebsen–Taylor Hand Function Test, and simple reaction times in the paretic hand that outlasted the stimulation period for at least 40 minutes. In contrast, sham stimulation during JTT practice did not show these same improvements [19]. The findings suggest such stimulation can improve skilled motor functions of the paretic hand in chronic stroke patients. The main risk with this technology is for skin burns from the direct electrical current but it is otherwise well tolerated.

Functional electrical stimulation

Direct electrical stimulation of the peripheral nervous system may also be a potential treatment for stroke survivors. This technique, known as functional electrical stimulation (FES), employs electrical stimulation to maintain and improve tone in weak muscles and increase muscle strength through peripheral mechanisms. In patients with pain and weakness in the upper limb and shoulder, stimulation of the posterior deltoid and supraspinatus muscles has been shown to be effective in reducing glenohumeral subluxation and decreasing shoulder pain following stroke. Furthermore, electrical stimulation of the wrist and finger extensors may enhance upper limb motor recovery in acute stroke patients and increases function.

Recently, a home-based stimulation-assisted training orthosis-stimulation system was developed that has led to increases in hand function in stroke patients. In contrast to the studies described above, peripheral nerve stimulation has been recently employed to induce central changes that might be beneficial for recovery following stroke. Somatosensory stimulation in the absence of muscle contraction has been shown to influence cortical reorganization. This has been demonstrated through the application of peripheral nerve stimulation to chronic stroke patients with upper limb hemiparesis and was tested in a randomized crossover design study involving a small number of patients. Pinch grip strength increased by 2.41 ± 0.74 Newtons ($P = 0.017$) following a 2-hour session of median nerve stimulation. Although no sham stimulation was used, patients reported improved ability to write and hold objects in the simulation group [20]. The authors believe the type of stimulation used in their design increased the amount of use-dependent plasticity as seen in chronic stroke patients when tested using transcranial magnetic stimulation (TMS), supporting the hypothesis that somatosensory input is able to drive plastic changes in the motor cortex following stroke.

Mental practice with motor imagery

Mental practice refers to a technique through which an individual repeatedly mentally rehearses an action or task without actually physically performing the action or task; the goal of the exercise is to improve actual physical performance of those actions or tasks. From a neuroplasticity standpoint, it would encourage repetition and goal direction.

EVIDENCE AT A GLANCE

In a review of six randomized controlled trials involving a total of 119 participants, the Cochrane group concluded that mental practice, when added to traditional physical rehabilitation treatments, improved upper extremity function compared with the use of traditional rehabilitation treatment alone. Furthermore, the combination of mental plus physical practice appears to be more effective in increasing upper extremity function than either treatment alone ($Z=3.48$, $P=0.0005$; standardized mean difference (SMD) 1.37; 95% confidence interval) [21]. Current evidence shows the improvements are measured in performance of real-life tasks appropriate to the upper limb (e.g. drinking from a cup, manipulating a door knob).

There is uncertainty surrounding the use of mental practice for stroke rehabilitation. The amount of mental practice and motor imagery that is needed to enhance traditional therapy has not been established. In a study comparing the amount of mental practice required with physical therapy, 60 minutes of mental practice optimized outcomes [22]. Subjects practiced for 20, 40, or 60 minutes and the largest increases in upper limb FM score were seen when volunteers engaged in 60 minutes of mental practice. Irrespective of mental practice duration, subjects administered mental practice exhibited markedly larger score changes on both the FM and ARAT than subjects not receiving mental practice; the authors concluded that that mental practice is beneficial to motor recovery following stroke regardless of the amount of time spent practicing [22]. Other studies affirming the benefit of mental practice with motor imagery have used 30 minutes duration of mental practice.

The phase of stroke recovery has implications for application of mental imagery therapy. The evidence-based Cochrane review found upper extremity functional improvement when mental imagery was used during the subacute and chronic stages of stroke recovery. A recent study found that mental practice did not have benefit compared to traditional therapy when applied to subjects less than 3 months from stroke onset. Larger

clinical trials are currently ongoing and should clarify the optimal timing and dosing of mental imagery therapy.

Virtual reality

Virtual reality (VR) is computer-based technology that allows users to interact with a multisensory simulated environment and receive "real-time" feedback on performance. VR leverages the principles of neuroplasticity to promote functional gains. In a VR environment a stroke survivor can perform repetitive, goal-directed movements while remaining engaged by playing "fun" games with varying levels of difficulty. Home-based gaming consoles such as Wii® and X-box Kinect® employ interactive VR technology and can provide immediate feedback, which is an important aspect of motor learning and can yield additional advantages over traditional forms of therapy. VR-based devices can be used at home and allow stroke survivors to potentially increase the dose of therapy compared to standard therapy resulting in improved functional outcomes.

A meta-analysis examining the effect of VR on upper extremity stroke rehabilitation found 11 of 12 studies with a significant benefit toward VR for the selected outcomes in arm function, most often measured using the upper limb Fugl–Myer scale [23]. Stroke survivors in the subacute and chronic phases of stroke were included in the analysis of five randomized controlled trials where the intervention was applied between 2 and 6 weeks. The pooled analysis of all five randomized controlled trials revealed the effect of VR on motor impairment as measured by Fugl–Myer was odds ratio (OR)=4.89 (95% CI, 1.31 to 18.3). In the remaining observational studies, there was a 14.7% (95% CI, 8.7–23.6%) improvement in motor impairment and a 20.1% (95% CI, 11.0–33.8%) improvement in motor function after VR [23].

In a meta-analysis included in the Cochran library involving 19 VR trials, improvement in upper extremity Fugl–Myer score and improvement in activities of daily living was seen [24]. Like the prior meta-analysis, the trials involved chronic stroke survivors between 30 and 83 years old. There was heterogeneity in length of intervention and types of the VR system employed. Whereas the first meta-analysis limited their review to the effect of VR to upper extremity function, the second meta-analysis explored the effect of VR on cognition and other global outcome measures. The meta-analysis found insufficient evidence to comment on the effect of VR therapy on markers of recovery from stroke such as grip strength or gait speed or quality of life, cognitive measures, or global activity measures. The other consistent findings among the studies reviewed were that use of VR technology for stroke rehabilitation is safe and feasible. Relatively few side-effects occur as a result of using the technology, with some reporting minor pain, headaches, or dizziness.

Stem cell therapy

Another potential therapeutic intervention is the utilization of stem cells as a treatment to enhance stroke recovery. As stem cells have the capacity to differentiate into various types of cells, it is believed that these cells, once transplanted, will develop into neurons and glial cells. In this way, stem cells will replace the tissue damaged from the stroke. However, it has been documented in the past decade that differentiation into neural cells is not absolutely necessary for the achievement of a beneficial outcome with this type of therapy. In fact, increasing evidence suggests that development of stems cells into neurons and glial cells may not be the major mechanism leading to recovery. First, the beneficial effect observed after transplantation appears too early for the differentiation and integration of cells into local circuits. Second, in some studies, although neuronal differentiation is seen, the degree of differentiation and integration of the transplanted cells do not correlate with functional outcome. As further support, a recent report has found that peripherally transplanted cells do not have to cross the blood–brain barrier at all to induce neurorestorative effects. In observational animal models, after endogenous stem cells migrate to an area of injury, they proliferate but then undergo apoptosis. It is likely that there are other mechanisms contributing to the therapeutic benefit of cell transplantation in stroke.

Currently, the cell types that have been tested for stroke recovery include embryonic stem cells (ESCs), adult-derived neural stem cells (NSCs), bone marrow or mesenchymal stem cells (BMSCs), and umbilical cord blood stem cells (UCBCs). In humans, the studies have considered implantation of stem cells and the safety of such requirements. The route of delivery of stem cells is still being investigated with delivery via intravenous, intra-arterial directly to the site of stroke via endovascular methods.

In addition to transplanting exogenous cells, another approach may be to recruit endogenous stem cells. Such endogenous stem cells have been seen in rat models of stroke where they reside in the subventricular zone. Stromal cell-derived factor-1 (SDF-1) and its receptor, CXC-chemokine receptor-4 (CXCR4) are important molecules in stem cell mobilization and migration. Erythropoietin (EPO) appears to also serve as a migration signaling molecule for stem cells. Therefore, an infusion of EPO can help promote migration of stem cells and may represent novel treatment options for stroke recovery. Stem cells have not been demonstrated in adult human brains to date but trials are ongoing to examine interventions that recruit these cells. The studies to date have investigated safety and practicality and changes in function and outcomes remain under investigation.

Research also focuses on the production of various trophic factors produced by stem cells. Such factors that have been shown to be a byproduct of stem cells include vascular endothelial growth factor (VEGF), fibroblast growth factor (FGF), glial cell-derived neurotrophic factor (GDNF), and brain-derived neurotrophic factor (BDNF). These factors play a role in synaptogenesis by promoting axon and/or dendritic growth. Conceptually, rather than replacing lost tissue, neural networks are restored by a rewiring process. Given the role of trophic factors in the mechanisms of stroke recovery, administration of these factors may be most efficacious. Some of these factors may be responsible for inducing migration of natural progenitor cells.

Summary

Recovery of function following stroke is a dynamic process. Despite the advances in prevention and acute treatment, stroke survivors will continue to need rehabilitation. Recovery begins as soon as the patient enters the health-care system. There is evidence that the choice of interventions to enhance poststroke recovery is dependent upon the phase of stroke recovery. An understanding of the mechanisms of stroke recovery has expedited the development of novel therapeutic techniques. New advances in imaging technology has been shown to provide prognostic information that augment traditional clinical exam. Future advances in the stroke recovery processes will be influenced by interventions such as TMS, tDCS, FES, VR, and MP, alone or in combination with traditional therapy. Although in their infancy, pharmacologic and stem cell therapies may hold promise for recovery of lost function in patients suffering from stroke.

Selected bibliography

1. Duncan PW, Lai SM, Keighley J. Defining post-stroke recovery: implications for design and interpretation of drug trials. *Neuropharmacology* 2000; **39**: 835–41.
2. Kwakkel G, Kollen B, Lindeman E. Understanding the pattern of functional recovery after stroke: facts and theories. *Restor Neurol Neurosci* 2004; **22**: 281–99.
3. Ottenbacher KJ, Jannell S. The results of clinical trials in stroke rehabilitation research. *Arch Neurol* 1993; **50**: 37–44.
4. Paolucci S, Antonucci G, Grasso MG, et al. Early versus delayed inpatient stroke rehabilitation: a matched comparison conducted in Italy. *Arch Phys Med Rehabil* 2000; **81**: 695–700.
5. Nijland RH, van Wegen EE, Harmeling-van der Wel BC, Kwakkel G. Presence of finger extension and shoulder abduction within 72 hours after stroke predicts functional recovery: early prediction of functional outcome after stroke: the EPOS cohort study. *Stroke* 2010; **41**: 745–50.
6. Zarahn E, Alon L, Ryan SL, et al. Prediction of motor recovery using initial impairment and fMRI 48 h poststroke. *Cereb Cortex* 2011; **21**: 2712–21.
7. DeVetten G, Coutts SB, Hill MD, et al. Acute corticospinal tract Wallerian degeneration is associated with stroke outcome. *Stroke* 2010; **41**: 751–6.
8. Cumming TB, Thrift AG, Collier JM, et al. Very early mobilization after stroke fast-tracks return to walking: further results from the phase II AVERT randomized controlled trial. *Stroke* 2011; **42**: 153–8.
9. Dromerick AW, Lang CE, Birkenmeier RL, et al. Very Early Constraint-Induced Movement during Stroke Rehabilitation (VECTORS): A single-center RCT. *Neurology* 2009; **73**: 195–201.
10. Zorowitz RD, Smout RJ, Gassaway JA, Horn SD. Neurostimulant medication usage during stroke rehabilitation: the Post-Stroke Rehabilitation Outcomes Project (PSROP). *Top Stroke Rehabil* 2005; **12**: 28–36.
11. Wolf SL, Winstein CJ, Miller JP, et al. Effect of constraint-induced movement therapy on upper extremity function 3 to 9 months after stroke: the EXCITE randomized clinical trial. *JAMA* 2006; **296**: 2095–104.
12. Berthier ML, Green C, Lara JP, et al. Memantine and constraint-induced aphasia therapy in chronic poststroke aphasia. *Ann Neurol* 2009; **65**: 577–85.
13. Welmer AK, von Arbin M, Widen Holmqvist L, Sommerfeld DK. Spasticity and its association with functioning and health-related quality of life 18 months after stroke. *Cerebrovasc Dis* 2006; **21**: 247–53.
14. Cramer SC, Nelles G, Benson RR, et al. A functional MRI study of subjects recovered from hemiparetic stroke. *Stroke* 1997; **28**: 2518–27.
15. Johansen-Berg H, Dawes H, Guy C, et al. Correlation between motor improvements and altered fMRI activity after rehabilitative therapy. *Brain* 2002; **125**: 2731–42.
16. Stinear CM, Barber PA, Smale P, et al. Functional potential in chronic stroke patients depends on corticospinal tract integrity. *Brain* 2007; **130**: 170–80.
17. Qiu M, Darling WG, Morecraft RJ, *et al.* White matter integrity is a stronger predictor of motor function than BOLD response in patients with stroke. *Neurorehabil Neural Rep* 2011; **25**: 275–84.
18. Khedr EM, Abo-Elfetoh N, Rothwell JC. Treatment of post-stroke dysphagia with repetitive transcranial magnetic stimulation. *Acta Neurol Scand* 2009; **119**: 155–61.
19. Hummel F, Cohen LG. Improvement of motor function with noninvasive cortical stimulation in a patient with chronic stroke. *Neurorehabil Neural Rep* 2005; **19**: 14–9.
20. Conforto AB, Kaelin-Lang A, Cohen LG. Increase in hand muscle strength of stroke patients after somatosensory stimulation. *Ann Neurol* 2002; **51**: 122–5.
21. Barclay-Goddard RE, Stevenson TJ, Poluha W, Thalman L. Mental practice for treating upper extremity deficits in individuals with hemiparesis after stroke. *Cochrane Database Syst Rev* 2011; (**5**): CD005950.

22. Page SJ, Dunning K, Hermann V, et al. Longer versus shorter mental practice sessions for affected upper extremity movement after stroke: a randomized controlled trial. *Clin Rehab* 2011; **25**: 627–37.

23. Saposnik G, Levin M, Outcome Research Canada (SORCan) Working Group. Virtual reality in stroke rehabilitation a meta-analysis and implications for clinicians. *Stroke* 2011; **42**: 1380–6.

24. Laver KE, George S, Thomas S, et al. Virtual reality for stroke rehabilitation. *Cochrane Database Syst Rev* 2011; (**9**): CD008349.

8

Telemedicine Networks and Remote Evaluation of the Acute Stroke Patient

Bart M. Demaerschalk, MD, MSc, FRCP(C)

Department of Neurology, Mayo Clinic, Phoenix, Arizona

Introduction

The availability of personnel and resources for acute stroke diagnosis and emergency management varies from one institution to another, across the United States, and around the globe [1]. Stroke centers are adequately equipped and sufficiently staffed, but unfortunately stroke centers represent only a minority of all hospitals. Forty percent of the United States population resides in counties without a hospital actively engaged in acute stroke care. Unfortunately, the level of expertise at a stroke center may not be available in nonspecialty designated hospitals that are located in some urban and in most rural communities [2]. Hence, there exists a major gap in availability of acute stroke care. Together, telemedicine technology and consultative stroke services are capable of overcoming this gap. Telemedicine is the use of electronic communication methods, such as the telephone, the Internet, and videoconferencing, to exchange medical information from one geographic site to another (Figure 8.1). Telestroke is the employment of telemedicine specifically for the diagnosis and treatment of ischemic and hemorrhagic stroke (Figure 8.2).

Strategies for telestroke network building

Summary of the evidence supporting telemedicine use in acute stroke diagnosis and management

The single best synthesis and summary of evidence for the use of telemedicine within stroke systems of care can be found in a scientific statement from the American Heart Association/American Stroke Association (AHA/ASA) published in 2009 [3]. This statement provided a comprehensive and evidence-based review of the scientific evidence supporting the use of telemedicine in acute stroke care delivery. The evidence is organized and presented within the context of the AHA Stroke Systems of Care framework and is classified according to the AHA/ASA methods of classifying the levels of evidence and classes of recommendations. The recommendations addressed telemedicine and teleradiology use in prehospital and emergency phases of acute stroke patient assessment and management. A summary of the recommendations applicable to this topic are presented in Table 8.1.

Utilization of thrombolysis for acute ischemic stroke may serve as a surrogate marker of a health-care institution's application of acute stroke management strategies. Despite financial incentives, the establishment of formal certification of primary stroke centers by the Joint Commission, the various statewide initiatives to standardize acute stroke care, and the AHA/ASA Get With The Guidelines campaign for stroke, national use of a thrombolytic agent for acute ischemic stroke has increased only modestly from approximately 0.9% in 1999, to 1.8–2.1% in 2004, to 3.4–5.2% in 2009 [4]. The factors still contributing to underutilization remain multifactorial and include public awareness of stroke symptoms and signs, 9-1-1 activation, geographic proximity to a stroke center, stroke specialist availability, immediate

Stroke, First Edition. Edited by Kevin M. Barrett and James F. Meschia.
© 2013 John Wiley & Sons, Ltd. Published 2013 by John Wiley & Sons, Ltd.

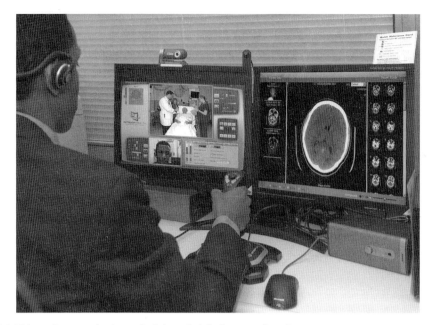

Figure 8.1 Telestroke consultation at hub hospital desktop workstation.

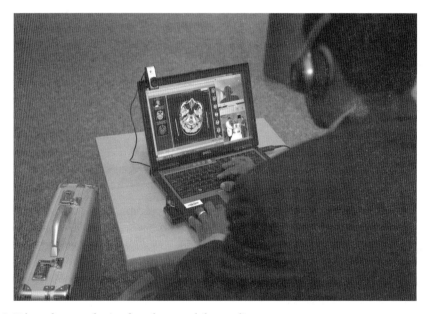

Figure 8.2 Telestroke consultation from laptop while traveling.

access to care, and complex diagnostic and therapeutic decision making. The rural to urban disparity regarding access to acute stroke resources, personnel, and therapies is immense. Eligible acute ischemic stroke patients in rural communities are ten times less likely to receive thrombolysis than those who inhabit metropolitan communities [5]. Telemedicine may increase access to stroke specialist expertise, especially for remote and rural communities but also for underserved urban

Table 8.1 AHA/ASA classification of recommendations and level of evidence for the use of telemedicine within stroke systems of care

No.	Recommendations	Class of recommendation, Level of evidence
1	The NIHSS-telestroke examination, when administered by a stroke specialist using high-quality videoconferencing, is recommended when an NIHSS bedside assessment by a stroke specialist is not immediately available for patients in the acute stroke setting, and this assessment is comparable to an NIHSS bedside assessment.	I, A
2	Teleradiology systems approved by the FDA (or equivalent organization) are recommended for timely review of brain CT scans in patients with suspected acute stroke.	I, A
3	Review of brain CT scans by stroke specialists or radiologists using teleradiology systems approved by the FDA (or equivalent organization) is useful for identifying exclusions for thrombolytic therapy in acute stroke patients.	I, A
4	When implemented within a telestroke network, teleradiology systems approved by the FDA (or equivalent organization) are useful in supporting rapid imaging interpretation in time for thrombolysis decision making.	I, B
5	It is recommended that a stroke specialist using high-quality videoconferencing provide a medical opinion in favor of or against the use of intravenous tPA in patients with suspected acute ischemic stroke when on-site stroke expertise is not immediately available.	I, B
6	Telephonic assessment for measuring functional disability after stroke is recommended when in-person assessment is impractical, the standardized rating instruments have been validated for telephonic use, and administration is by trained personnel using a structured interview.	I, B
7	Compared with traditional bedside evaluation and use of intravenous tPA, the safety and efficacy of intravenous tPA administration based solely on telephone consultation without CT interpretation via teleradiology are not well established.	IIb, C
8	Prehospital telephone-based contact between emergency medical personnel and stroke specialists for screening and consent can be effective in facilitating enrollment into hyperacute neuroprotective trials.	IIa, B

Data from Schwamm LH, Holloway RG, Amarenco P, et al. A review of the evidence for the use of telemedicine within stroke systems of care. A scientific statement from the AHA/ASA. *Stroke* 2009; **40**: 2616–34.

environments. Telemedicine may be implemented within a stroke system of care model to address these deficiencies in care delivery. One way to reduce the time interval from symptom onset to assessment and to treatment would be to provide remote assistance to emergency medical services (EMS) providers as they attempt to identify potential stroke patients and transport them to designated stroke centers. Prehospital telemedicine at the stroke scene or in a ground or air ambulance transport environment may increase diagnostic accuracy, help distinguish between stroke and stroke mimics, provide earlier stroke team resource mobilization, increase appropriate triage, enable neuroprotective agents to be administered, and provide a seamless continuity of care from prehospital to hospital environments [6]. Unfortunately, published applications have had unacceptably low frame rates and broad utilization to large fleets of EMS vehicles is not yet practical. At the time of AHA/ASA evidence review, there were insufficient data to support a recommendation for prehospital EMS telestroke applications. In the interim, the concept of seamless integrated stroke telemedicine systems of care was proposed as a

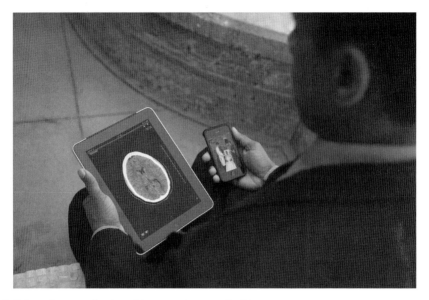

Figure 8.3 Telestroke consultation with smartphone and tablet.

potential solution for acute stroke care delivery delays and inefficiencies. Prehospital real-time cellular video phone assessment of the National Institutes of Health Stroke Scale (NIHSS) in patients with acute stroke was determined to be feasible, reliable, and timely [7]. Remote assessment of NIHSS using the iPhone 4 FaceTime function compared with bedside assessment revealed excellent inter-rater reliability [8] (Figure 8.3). A new stroke support system using a mobile device (Smartphone) for diagnostic image display and treatment of stroke (i-Stroke system) includes a Tweet function that simultaneously alerts and virtually unites every contributing stroke team member around the patient and a synchronized chronological time line that begins with symptom onset. The system enables simultaneous communication among several team members and results in significant time savings on decision making. The Tweet function permits stroke team members to instantly enter and transmit comments about clinical images, neuroimaging, and related diagnostic data [9].

Strategies for funding the development of a telestroke network

Various strategies are available to fund the development of a telestroke network, as given in Table 8.2.

Table 8.2 Start-up telestroke network funding options

Telemedicine grants
Research grants
Benefactor funding
Spoke subsidization
Hub subsidization
Hub and spoke subsidization
Spoke subscription-based revenue stream
Health insurance reimbursement (government and nongovernment insurers)
Combination of above

Economic sustainability, cost effectiveness, and the status of reimbursement for telestroke

Economic vulnerability continues to threaten the sustainability of telestroke networks. The ASA has recommended that new models and codes for reimbursement of telestroke services be developed to reflect the increased upfront costs to providers and reduced long-term health-care costs to insurers [10]. The ASA recommends that increased reimbursement under Medicare for thrombolysis delivery in the United States under stroke thrombolysis Diagnosis-Related Group (DRG) (MS-DRG 61 to 63) should be available to hospitals that supervise the initiation of thrombolysis via telestroke and then accept these patients in transfer for admission to the hub hospital (drip and ship). The ASA has encouraged Medicare and private payers to adopt similar telestroke reimbursement policies to apply uniformly to both rural and urban spoke hospital environments. On-call stipends and other incentives are recommended to encourage participation by vascular neurologists.

Miley et al. assembled a representative budget for a telestroke network, including costs associated with neurology personnel, coordinators, managers, information technologists, administrators, telemedicine platform equipment, supplies, laptop cameras, headsets with microphones, broadband wireless cards, efax subscriptions, travel expenses, training, and overhead [11]. The start-up and first year of operation costs for a multihub network serving 35 rural spoke hospitals was $2.5 million. On average, the annual cost associated with adding a new rural spoke hospital to a telestroke network is $46,000 but can vary from less than $10,000 to more than $200,000 per year, dependent upon the size of hospital, volume of stroke consultations, and sophistication of telemedicine equipment selected [12].

Obtaining direct revenue from insurance payers for telestroke consultations sufficient to sustain a network is difficult. Medicare will only reimburse for telemedicine consultations that involve live two-way audio–video communication between patient and hub vascular neurologist and only when the spoke is located in an eligible underserved geographic locale. Medicare defines these eligible regions as rural health professional shortage areas and counties not classified as a metropolitan statistical area. Jon Linkous, CEO, American Telemedicine Association, emphasized the availability of category III Current Procedural Terminology (CPT) codes for critical care telemedicine services, 0188T and 0189T, but notes that national coverage and payment policies for category III CPT codes do not yet exist and payments may vary among public and commercial payers [13]. Linkous drew attention to what's ahead. Recent federal action has resulted in added codes for Medicare telehealth, and Medicare privileging rules and rural health program changes are pending.

> ## EVIDENCE AT A GLANCE
>
> In 2010, Demaerschalk et al. conducted a systematic review of the published literature analyzing cost effectiveness or cost savings associated with use of thrombolysis, stroke centers, and telemedicine programs for acute ischemic stroke [14]. No cost-effectiveness studies for stroke centers or telemedicine programs were identified. The authors concluded that more high-quality, current cost-effectiveness research for stroke centers, care networks, and telemedicine was needed to inform treatment decisions and resource utilization.

Fortunately, Nelson et al. conducted the first US cost-effectiveness analysis of telestroke in the treatment of acute ischemic stroke [15]. Two-way audio–video technology linking a single hub hospital of stroke specialists to a network of eight remote emergency departments and their stroke patients was compared to usual care (i.e. remote emergency departments without telestroke consultation or stroke expertise). A decision analytic model was developed for both 90-days and lifetime horizons. Model inputs included both costs and clinical consequences. Quality adjusted life years (QALYs) gained were combined with costs to generate incremental cost-effectiveness ratios (ICERs). In the base case analysis, compared to usual care, telestroke resulted in an ICER of $108,363/QALY in the 90-day horizon and $2449/QALY in the lifetime horizon. Therefore, authors concluded that telestroke appeared cost effective. Subsequent telestroke economic research focused on the perspective of the hub and spoke hospitals in a network [16]. Compared with no network, a network model resulted in more patients treated with IV thrombolysis, more patients transferred for endovascular management, and more patients discharged home independently. The telestroke network cost less, overall, and was more effective than no network. With increased spoke-to-hub transfer rates, the hub experiences greater cost savings while the spokes bear higher costs. Within networks designed to reduce spoke-to-hub transfer rates, the spokes experience greater cost

Table 8.3 AHA/ASA recommendations for implementing telemedicine within the stroke systems of care

No.	Recommendation
1	Telestroke systems should be deployed to supplement existing personnel and resources in instances when local on-site acute stroke expertise are insufficient to provide around-the-clock coverage for a hospital.
2	Rules, principles, and contractual agreements should govern the services and interactions between telestroke provider (hub hospital) and recipient (spoke hospital). Contracts should address: assignment of costs, compliance with government boundaries and noncompete relationships, medicolegal risk, malpractice coverage, sharing of protected health information, administration, licensing and credentialing, reimbursement for professional fees, and roles and responsibilities.
3	Patients or surrogate should be informed of the request for a telestroke consultation and should grant permission. Medical advice and documentation should be provided during a telestroke consultation in a manner similar to an on-site face-to-face interaction.
4	Telemedicine technology vendors should adhere to widely accepted industry standards.
5	Telemedicine technology should be easy to use for hub and spoke. The network must have a mechanism and plan for technology failure and a fail-safe solution when a timely repair is not realistic.
6	New models and codes for telemedicine reimbursement, applicable to telestroke, should be developed.
7	Mechanisms for national or multistate licensure limited to telemedicine practice should be adopted by state medical boards. Streamlined credentialing and privileging avenues ought to be promoted, whenever they exist.
8	The use of telemedicine should be deployed within all stroke systems of care components to eliminate geographic disparities in care that may occur as a result of limited resources or personnel.
9	Prior to establishing telestroke network connectivity, hospitals should engage key stakeholders, including, at a minimum, physicians, nurses, and allied health staff in emergency medicine, neurology, neurosurgery, hospitalist medicine, radiology, administration, and IT.

Data from Schwamm LH, Audebert HJ, Amarenco P, et al. Recommendations for the implementation of telemedicine within stroke systems of care: A policy statement from the AHA/ASA. *Stroke* 2009; **40**: 2635–60.

savings while the hub bears higher costs. Health economic research, such as this, may help networks develop viable and sustainable business plans.

Fundamentals of telestroke networks

Implementation of telemedicine within stroke systems of care

Please see Table 8.3, summarizing general recommendations regarding the implementation of telemedicine within stroke systems of care.

Incorporating evidence-based practice guidelines and care pathways into a telestroke network

Organizations providing telestroke services and organizations receiving telestroke services should collaboratively adopt and apply evidence-based stroke practice guidelines to every level of the interaction, from prehospital care through to rehabilitation and reintegration into the community (Figure 8.4). Ideally, the AHA/ASA guidelines, practice parameters, and scientific statements applicable to stroke should be readily available on-line to hub and spoke providers and serve as the substrate for collaborative telestroke in-service training and continuing medical education. Spoke site visits to review evidence and guidelines, building or updating evidence-based stroke order sets and care pathways and algorithms, in-service training for spoke personnel, and sharing best practices hub to spoke and spoke to spoke are all potential ways to transmit "best evidence" and to incorporate evidence-based practice into the hub and spoke telestroke dynamic.

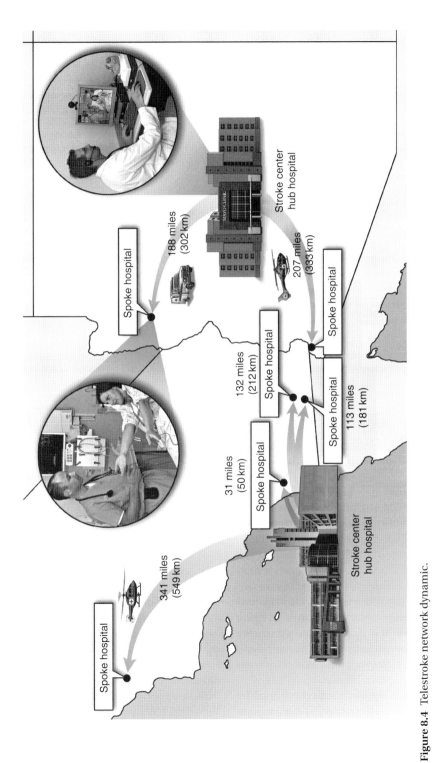

Figure 8.4 Telestroke network dynamic.

Table 8.4 Telestroke stakeholder representatives and champions at hub and spoke hospitals

Hub hospital	Spoke hospital
Director (e.g. Vascular Neurologist)	Director (e.g. Emergency Physician)
Program manager	Program manager
Program education coordinator	Program education coordinator
Teleneurologists	Emergency physicians
Teleneurosurgeons	Hospitalists
Teleneuroradiologists	Intensivists
Teleneurointerventionalists	Local neurologist(s) if applicable
Information technologists	Information technologists
Nurse practitioners or physician assistants	Midlevel providers, emergency medicine
Lawyer	Lawyer
Administrative assistant	Radiologist (or teleradiologist)
Billing and coding analyst	Laboratory
Financial analyst	Emergency nurses
Operations administrator	Emergency medical services (EMS)
Contracts advisor	Contracts advisor
Marketing analyst	Quality representatives
Grant writer	Radiology technologists
Health policy and administration advisor	Billing and coding analyst
Research coordinator	Research coordinators
Public affairs representative	Public affairs representative

Table 8.5 Conceptual framework for telestroke network adoption

Technological context	Environmental context	Organizational context	Project planning context
Compatibility	Government support	Management support	Team skills
Relative advantage	Competitive pressure	Technical knowledge	Resources
Supplier support	Insurer support	Internal need	User participation

Engaging stakeholders

Please see Table 8.4 listing potential stakeholders with which to engage for telestroke development. A champion representing each category or division or department serves well to ensure that the stakeholders remain engaged during the planning and execution phases of telestroke.

Administrative infrastructure

Liu et al. have developed a conceptual framework which illustrates the key factors influencing telestroke network adoption. The authors have organized the 12 factors under four contextual headings [17] (Table 8.5).

Successful telestroke teams are generally led by a medical director who partners with a program manager or operations administrator. Please refer to Table 8.4 for other key team roles.

★ TIPS AND TRICKS

Every telestroke program should develop a vision, build a core infrastructure, and assemble a core team. Part of the team's assignment will be to construct standardized policies, procedures, consents, checklists, instructions, and a manual of operations.

The program vision may have different definitions of success, for example optimizing patient outcomes, improving access, financial metrics (net operating income), patient volume (numbers of patients assessed), establishing higher levels of care, community outreach, and research.

Telestroke technology options

Telemedicine has been broadly defined as the use of telecommunications technologies to provide medical information and services. Telestroke is the use of telemedicine in the form of videoconferencing (VTC) to support acute stroke intervention. Dedicated, high-quality, interactive, bidirectional audio–visual systems coupled with the use of teleradiology for remote review of neuroimaging constitutes VTC telestroke systems. High-quality videoconferencing (HQ-VTC) methodology allows the patient, family, bedside health-care providers, and remote providers to see and hear each other using remote-control cameras with pan-tilt-zoom capabilities. Telemedicine systems should meet certain minimum quality standards for HQ-VTC, including transmission rates and algorithms of sufficient quality to support more than 20 frames per second of bidirectional synchronized audio and video at a resolution capable of being accurately displayed on monitors of 13 inches or larger. These parameters reflect the consensus expert opinion of the AHA/ASA writing group. Common intermediate format (CIF) is used to standardize the horizontal and vertical resolutions in pixels in video signals, commonly used in HQ-VTC systems. CIF defines a video sequence with resolution of 352×288 at a frame rate of 30 frames per second in full color. Earlier systems used dedicated high-speed telecommunications lines, usually integrated services digital network (ISDN) lines, at rates of 256 to 384 kilobits per second to achieve CIF transmission. Recent developments in quality of private fiberoptic networks and public Internet providers and different vendors using different video processing, numeric statements about transmission rates may no longer reflect comparable image quality across vendors. Instead, it may be better to focus on visual resolution and latency (CIF standards) which are properties that will remain meaningful even as technology evolves. Teleradiology is the ability to obtain radiographic images at one location and transmit them remotely to another location for diagnostic and consultative purposes. The American College of Radiology published standards for digital imaging and communications in medicine (DICOM) and for teleradiology applications. The Joint Commission is involved in the appraisal and credentialing of teleradiology systems.

See Table 8.6 giving vendors of telemedicine technology.

Table 8.6 Vendors of telemedicine technology

Telemedicine cart vendor	Head office location
BF Technologies/ MedAccess	San Diego, California
Emerge.MD, Inc	Phoenix, Arizona
Global Med	Scottsdale, Arizona
InTouch Health	Santa Barbara, California
Lifesize	Austin, Texas
Polycom	Pleasanton, California
REACH	Augusta, Georgia
Remote Meeting Technologies	Melville, New York
Specialists on Call	Westlake Village, California
Tandberg	New York, New York
Vidyo	Hackensack, New Jersey

Metrics to track performance, outcomes, and quality of a telestroke network

Schwamm et al. recommend that every telestroke network hub and spoke hospital participate in the collection of applicable state or national stroke quality measures. At a minimum, continuous quality improvement activities should include assessment of adoption and use of technology, rates of technical and human failure related to the system, and needs for training and maintaining competency. The results of quality, performance, and outcome metrics should be shared across the network. The Joint Commission has published telemedicine requirements for hospital and critical access hospital accreditation programs to ensure that care, treatment, and services provided through contractual agreements are provided safely and effectively.

Telestroke networks

Silva et al. conducted an environmental scan of telestroke programs in the United States, attempting to locate any potential programs operating since the year 2000 [18]. A dedicated project analyst contacted all identified programs, interviewed respondents in-depth, and collected on-line survey data assessing structural and functional aspects of the programs. The results demonstrated a total of 100 possible telestroke programs existed in 43 states. Thirty-eight percent of the programs agreed to participate in the research. The top three clinical needs met by the telestroke programs were emergency department consultation (100%), patient triage (84%), and in-patient teleconsultation (46%). The median telestroke program duration of operation was 891 days. Most (95%) of the programs used two-way, real-time, interactive video plus teleradiology in their consultation algorithms. Dedicated telemedicine software was used by 44% of the programs to capture and save consultations. The mean number of spokes per hub increased from 2007 to 2009 (3.78 vs. 7.60; P <0.05; maximum 28). In over half of the networks, more than 80% of the spoke sites were small rural hospitals with fewer than 100 beds. Reimbursement for telestroke was limited: none (43%), private insurance (30%), Medicare (27%), Medicaid (22%), and Tricare (5%) [18]. The three key factors driving development of telestroke networks were to provide a community benefit (97%), to improve clinical outcomes (92%), and to improve care processes (76%). Networks identified inability to obtain licenses (28%), insufficient funds (28%), and lack of reimbursement (19%) as the three most significant obstacles for telestroke practice.

See Table 8.7 for telestroke networks reported capacity to increase thrombolysis administration.

Overcoming challenges to sustain a telestroke network

Identifying and overcoming obstacles (licensing, credentialing, privileging, medicolegal, financial, and reimbursement issues)

Multiple regulatory issues have been identified as barriers to implementing and sustaining telemedicine programs. Survey research results revealed an overall consensus that licensing out-of-state physicians, concern over malpractice liability, credentialing for medical staff privileges at individual facilities, and reimbursement limitations are all significant impediments for telemedicine networks [19].

Most states have specific licensing provisions for telemedicine. The physical location of the patient is generally accepted as the location at which medicine is being practiced, as opposed to the physical location of the telemedicine physician provider. In most instances, individual states require a full, unrestricted medical license before telemedicine practice is authorized. For practical purposes, an individual telestroke provider would require a medical license for each and every state of network

practice in order to comply. The requirement of a license for every state poses a significant administrative burden upon telestroke network providers and their managers. The creation of a national (or even multistate) telemedicine license would be a logical solution to encourage telestroke network expansion. However, the licensing rules vary state by state. Some states have introduced specific telemedicine licenses (Alabama, Montana, Minnesota, Ohio, Oklahoma, Oregon, Texas, and Tennessee) or special-purpose telemedicine licenses (Nevada), some states require full licenses to conduct telemedicine care (California, Florida, and New York) with exceptions for consultation only, and other states are still exploring regulation of telemedicine. Mutual recognition of telemedicine licenses would be highly desirable.

Traditionally, the requirement for every telestroke provider to undergo independent credentialing and privileging at a hub hospital and at every spoke hospital placed a very high administrative burden upon hospital staff. Fortunately, Centers for Medicare and Medicaid Services (CMS) have introduced a new rule for the credentialing and privileging of telemedicine physicians and practitioners which went into effect on July 5th, 2011. The Medicare conditions of participation previously required the governing body of a hospital to make all privileging decisions based on the recommendation of the hospital's medical staff after the medical staff had thoroughly reviewed the credentials of practitioners applying for privileges. This requirement was applied regardless of whether the services were to be provided on-site at the hospital or through a tele-communications system. The new CMS rule allows the hospital receiving telemedicine services to rely upon credentialing and privileging information from the hospital providing the telemedicine services (credentialing and privileging by proxy). The new rule has effectively reduced the administrative burden, at hub and spoke, associated with telestroke provider credentialing and privileging.

Legal barriers to telestroke practice also exist. The federal antikickback statute makes illegal any arrangement where one purpose is to offer, solicit, or pay anything of value in return for a referral for treatment. Whether or not the provision of subsidized or free telemedicine equipment or services violates the statute has been an issue under review and debate. An incentive for telestroke network

Table 8.7 Reported thrombolysis amongst telestroke networks

Telestroke network study (reference)	Proportion of telestroke alert consultation patients reported to receive thrombolysis
STRokE DOC (Meyer et al. 2008)	28%
Partners TeleStroke (Schwamm et al. 2004)	25%
CO-DOC (Fanale personal communication)	22%
Maryland (LaMonte et al. 2003)	24%
STRokE DOC AZ TIME (Demaerschalk et al. 2010)	30%
STARR (Demaerschalk et al. 2009)	27%
Mayo Clinic Telestroke (Demaerschalk unpublished data)	19%
REACH (Hess et al. 2005)	15%
Ontario Telestroke Network (Waite et al. 2006)	31%
Michigan Stroke Network (http://www.michiganstrokenetwork.com)	18%
TEMPiS (Schwab et al. 2007)	10-fold increase in thrombolysis
Finnish Telestroke (Sairanen et al. 2011)	58%
University of Utah (Majersik personal communication)	27%
REACH-MUSC (Lazaridis et al. 2011)	36% (of patients with NIHSS >3)

From Meyer BC, Demaerschalk BM. Telestroke network fundamentals. *J Stroke Cerebrovasc Dis* 2012; **21**: 521–9, with adaptations and modifications.

References:

Meyer BC, Raman R, Hemmen T, et al. Efficacy of site-independent telemedicine in the STRokE DOC trial: a randomised, blinded, prospective study. *Lancet Neurol* 2008; **7**: 787–95.

Schwamm LH, Rosenthal ES, Hirshberg A, et al. Virtual TeleStroke support for the emergency department evaluation of acute stroke. *Acad Emerg Med* 2004; **11**: 1193–7.

LaMonte MP, Bahouth MN, Hu P, et al. Telemedicine for acute stroke: triumphs and pitfalls. *Stroke* 2003; **34**: 725–8.

Demaerschalk B, Bobrow BJ, Raman R, et al. Stroke team remote evaluation using a digital observation camera in Arizona: the initial Mayo clinic experience trial. *Stroke* 2010; **41**: 1251–8.

Demaerschalk B, Miley ML, Kiernan TE, et al. Stroke telemedicine. *Mayo Clin Proc* 2009; **84**: 53–64 (Review). Erratum in: *Mayo Clin Proc* 2010; **85**: 400.

Hess DC, Wang S, Hamilton W, et al. REACH: clinical feasibility of a rural telestroke network. *Stroke* 2005; **36**: 2018–20.

Waite K, Silver F, Jaigobin C, et al. Telestroke: a multi-site, emergency-based telemedicine service in Ontario. *J Telemed Telecare* 2006; **12**: 141–5.

Schwab S, Vatankhah B, Kukla C, et al. Long-term outcome after thrombolysis in telemedical stroke care. *Neurology* 2007; **69**: 898–903.

Sairanen T, Soinila S, Nikkanen M, et al. Two years of Finnish Telestroke: thrombolysis at spokes equal to that at the hub. *Neurology* 2011; **76**: 1145–52.

Lazaridis C, Desantis SM, Jauch EC, et al. Telestroke in South Carolina. *J Stroke Cerebrovasc Dis* 2011, in press.

affiliate hospitals to refer to one another may exist, inherent to their regional connectedness. To the degree that a hub hospital bears the majority of the costs, and to the extent that access to the hub hospital by remote physicians results in referrals, an antikickback remuneration potential may exist. Fortunately, the Department of Health and Human Services (Re: OIG Advisory Opinion 11–12) believes that it is unlikely that the Office of the Inspector General would impose antikickback sanctions upon hub and spoke telestroke network work arrange-

ments given that the following conditions are met: there are no prespecified requirements to refer or transfer patients, there are no emergency medicine physician compensations, the overall telestroke network goal is to reduce spoke-to-hub transfers, the spoke patients benefit from expert assessment and treatment that might not otherwise be provided, the participating spoke hospitals benefit from enhanced health education and training, and that the telestroke network is unlikely to increase the overall cost to federal health-care programs.

Ensuring the privacy and security of information transmitted via telemedicine systems are vital legal requirements. When medical information is being transmitted, stored, or retrieved in digitized form, privacy and security threats exist. Unauthorized access and disclosure of electronic medical records must be prevented. Privacy and security can be maintained by Secure Sockets Layer (SSL) conditional access, data encryption, intruder alerts, and access logging and reporting. Virtual private networks (VPN) can provide encrypted connections over the internet. Multiple security features integrated into the technology ensures Health Information Portability and Accountability Act (HIPAA) compliance for virtual telestroke consultations.

In reference to medical liability, there is no specific evidence to suggest that providing telemedicine consultations increases the risk of malpractice claims compared with providing direct face-to-face consultations for the treatment of patients with acute stroke [1]. From the telestroke consultant perspective, the duties, responsibilities, and obligations are not different from those present during an in-person physician-to-patient relationship. The consultant's duty is similar for virtual and direct episodes of acute stroke care. The ASA recommends that medical advice be provided during a telestroke consultation in a manner similar to that which occurs during a face-to-face encounter. From the referring emergency medicine physician and spoke hospital perspective, historically the largest cause of malpractice accusations in stroke is failure to consider or to provide thrombolysis. Since telestroke networks within established stroke systems of care increase safe, appropriate, and effective use of thrombolysis in stroke, they are likely to safeguard against malpractice vulnerabilities.

★ TIPS AND TRICKS

It is advisable for telestroke providers to carry adequate malpractice coverage, perform timely consultations, communicate effectively, seek consent for the telemedicine consultation and for thrombolysis when applicable, and document assessment and decision making in an effort to reduce adverse patient outcomes and to minimize risk and consequences of litigation.

Financial barriers remain major obstacles to any telestroke network operation because of both the high up-front capital expenditure and the lack of reimbursement opportunities. While many professional societies lobby to gain support for physician reimbursement for telemedicine, the CMS has only recently established a telemedicine code (effective January 2010). Unfortunately, the code is not broadly applicable to all telestroke network environments. CMS requires that two-way, real-time, interactive audio–video telemedicine be conducted and that the referring site (spoke hospital at which the CMS beneficiary is located) must be in either a rural health professional shortage area or a county that is not included in a metropolitan statistical area in order for the work to be eligible for reimbursement. Each state has its own regulations for private payers. Regulation concerning the issue of mandatory telemedicine reimbursement exists only for California, Colorado, Hawaii, Kentucky, Louisiana, Maine, New Hampshire, Oregon, Oklahoma, Texas, and Virginia. There is potential for telestroke spoke hospitals to improve their reimbursement if the become increasingly engaged in the practice of telemedicine-aided thrombolysis and post-thrombolysis care for acute stroke patients. Unfortunately, an entirely unresolved reimbursement barrier occurs following a telestroke consultation which results in the provision of thrombolytic in the spoke hospital emergency department followed by transfer of the patient to the hub hospital. In these instances (drip and ship), neither the spoke nor hub facility is eligible to bill the higher MS-DRG codes (MS-DRG 61-63) associated with thrombolytic administration. Telestroke network cost-effectiveness research conducted from the hub and spoke perspective submitted for presentation at the 2012 Annual Meeting of the American Academy of Neurology revealed that compared to no network, a single hub and seven spoke hospital set-up resulted in 45 more patients treated with intravenous thrombolysis, 20 more patients treated with endovascular stroke therapies, and five additional discharges home with independence per 1000 acute ischemic stroke patients per year [16]. Across a span of spoke-to-hub transfer rates from 0% (all telestroke patients admitted to spoke) to 100% (all telestroke patients transferred to hub),

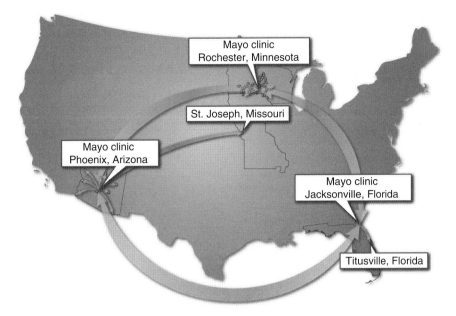

Figure 8.5 Mayo Clinic Telestroke Network.

incremental cost savings of $550,000 to $6,000 for the network as a whole, an incremental cost burden of $1,500,000 to a cost savings of $3,500,000 for the hub hospital, and an incremental cost savings of $300,000 to a cost burden of $500,000 for each spoke hospital. Expressed differently, as the spoke-to-hub transfer rate increases the network as a whole faces a reduction in cost savings associated with telestroke activity, the hub hospital benefits with a steady rise in cost savings, but at the expense of the spoke hospital which faces a reduction in cost savings (and instead bears rising incremental costs). The key factors that influence the telestroke network cost-effectiveness exchange are thrombolysis administration, spoke-to-hub transfer rate, and endovascular interventions for stroke.

Different dynamics and relationships may exist between hub hospitals and spoke hospitals in any given network and even between any two facilities within a network (Figure 8.5). Some smaller and/or poorly resourced and staffed hospitals (e.g. <100-bed facilities) may be capable of effective drip and ship thrombolysis under telemedicine guidance followed by transfer to the hub hospital stroke center [20,21].

EVIDENCE AT A GLANCE

The safety and early outcomes of patients treated with thrombolysis for acute ischemic stroke by the drip and ship method were compared to patients directly treated at a stroke center. Seventy-two percent were treated within 3 hours of symptom onset, median NIHSS score was 9.5, the median door-to-needle time was 85 minutes, the in-hospital mortality was 10.7%, the symptomatic intracranial hemorrhage rate was 6%, 30% had an early excellent outcome, and 75% were discharged home or qualified for acute in-patient rehabilitation.

These outcomes were not statistically different from those for stroke patients thrombolysed directly at a stroke center. In this small retrospective study, drip and ship approach did not appear to compromise safety.

Other larger and better equipped and staffed hospitals (e.g. 200-bed facilities) may have the personnel and resources to admit stroke patients following thrombolysis (drip and admit or drip and keep). Criteria have been proposed to aid in the decision making regarding the necessity of transferring a stroke patient from spoke to hub, but these decisions are still best made patient by patient, stroke by stroke, taking into account the patient's clinical syndrome characteristics, available spoke hospital personnel and resources, necessary diagnostic tests, the medical and surgical management being proposed, proximity of the hub hospital, and the hub hospital's capabilities. Several proposed criteria that may warrant consideration of transfer to a higher level of care may include: high NIH Stroke Scale score, large hemispheric infarction, intracranial hemorrhage with intraventricular extension, requirement for endovascular revascularization with thrombolysis or mechanical devices, hemicraniectomy for malignant hemispheric infarction with edema, mass effect, and herniation, posterior fossa decompression for hemorrhage or infarction, extracranial cervical carotid artery revascularization by endarterectomy or angioplasty and stenting, craniotomy for hematoma evacuation, ventricular drainage for hydrocephalus, clipping or coiling for intracranial aneurysms, or embolization or surgery for arteriovenous malformations.

Tips and tools for sustaining a telestroke network

The major determinants of a successful hub and spoke telestroke network are the health-care professionals and their relationships. The personnel and effective interactions between hub and spoke are more important than the telemedicine technology. Effective telestroke relationships successfully fulfill the clinical and economic needs of hub and spoke hospitals and health-care institutions, and require ongoing and repeated hub–spoke contact (both in-person as well as virtual connections). See Table 8.4 for key telestroke network representatives, stakeholders, and champions.

Getting buy-in from referring physicians, administrative leadership, and telemedicine providers

Gaining the attention of prospective spoke hospital leadership is easier with published evidence of telestroke safety, efficacy, and cost effectiveness. Strategies for presenting telestroke opportunities to hospital officials may include: letters, emails, pamphlets, websites, word-of-mouth, administrator to administrator dialogue, testimonials from satisfied patients, spoke hospitals, doctors, benefactors, community leaders, and politicians.

> ### ☆ TIPS AND TRICKS
>
> Effective planning prior to travel and spoke site visits may include gaining a clear understanding of a prospective spoke hospital's strengths and weakness regarding stroke resources, care, and outcomes, its objectives regarding acute stroke care (stroke patient retention versus transfer), and the perspectives of key stakeholders. Administrative and clinical leaders may be more receptive to considering a telestroke solution if a compelling clinical and economic case is established and presented.

Maintaining effective relationships between spoke emergency medicine physicians and hub neurologists is of paramount importance for the operations of a telestroke network. Several strategies to strengthen the consultative relationship include: providing a 1-800 telestroke hotline which provides a direct connection to a dedicated available neurology provider 24/7/365, simple pragmatic telestroke hotline eligibility criteria, a telemedicine algorithm that is easy to follow, a quick response time (<10 minutes), accepting all referrals without questioning or challenging, working effectively with bedside emergency nursing personnel so as not to unnecessarily hold up the emergency physician from evaluating other patients, evaluating urgently, collaborating with emergency personnel on diagnosis and the treatment plan, communicating effectively with the patient, family, nurse, and physician, documenting, and facilitating transfers whenever indicated.

For hub hospital telestroke providers, incentives, salary increase, on-call stipend, time-off compensation, access to technology, provision of new skills, participation in research trials and publications, and appearing in media presentations may all assist with fair compensation for any incremental work which may be associated with participating in a telestroke network.

Telestroke staff education

Education and orientation are necessary for new staff at both hub and spoke hospitals. At the hub hospital, each new telestroke provider will require instruction on telemedicine technology, trouble shooting, algorithm for consultation, and on spoke hospital characteristics pertaining to capacity, resources, personnel, and transfer. Educating a new spoke hospital and all of its personnel is as critical but more time consuming. Spoke hospital staff education will likely be targeted to include EMS providers, emergency nurses and physicians, hospitalists, intensivists, nurses, pharmacists, laboratory technologists, and radiology technicians.

★ TIPS AND TRICKS

Short, tailored, focused educational messages targeted to individual provider groups at a spoke hospital are more effective, efficient, and respectful of the providers' competing responsibilities and duties than a long one-size-fits-all lecture approach.

Examples of commonly used education modules include the NIH Stroke Scale assessment, the general neurological examination, central nervous system anatomy, a step-by-step telestroke consultation algorithm, technical trouble shooting, review of any relevant stroke guidelines, order-sets, and pathways.

Keeping hub and spoke partners engaged; how to combat telemedicine fatigue

Telestroke hub hospitals, spoke facilities, and the networks which joins them are all vulnerable to fatigue and a resultant drop in consultation rate and results, clinical and economic. The excitement and satisfaction of new technology, a new mode of neurological practice, the new professional relationships which develop, and the new extended reach of expertise, which all come from initiating a hub and spoke telestroke network, may wane and give way to frustration over incremental workload and any of several telestroke barriers which remain. Fatigue amongst telestroke referring doctors and providers is a reality amongst networks. Strategies that may combat the fatigue element include: telestroke network newsletters, tracking and broadcasting metrics, setting targets, rewarding successful personnel and sites, introducing novel technology, participating in stroke research trials, team celebrations, annual conferences, favorable media attention, conducting mock telestroke alerts, participating in research publications, hub-to-spoke continuing medical education and training, spoke-to-spoke sharing of best practices, utilizing telemedicine for training and mentoring residents and fellows at hub and spoke facilities, expanding telestroke coverage to new spoke sites or expanding telemedicine services to other medical and surgical disciplines, and conducting spoke site visits.

Conclusion

Telemedicine, applied to emergency stroke care, has been demonstrated to extend the reach of clinical stroke providers. This allows stroke teams to provide care in more than one location, overcome geographic barriers, reduce the urban-to-rural disparity gap, and improve the quality and timeliness of acute stroke diagnosis and treatment. The result is improved patient outcomes combined with reduced health-care expenditures. These exciting propositions are tempered by the realization that current telemedicine technology, its application, and broad implementation still require refinements in order to have more affordable, adaptable, smaller, mobile, portable, and universally applicable devices. Independent of the technology, telemedicine systems face other obstacles, including licensing, credentialing, and privileging of telemedicine providers within and across states, establishing sustainable business models, and adequate government and nongovernment insurance reimbursement.

Selected bibliography

1. Demaerschalk BM. Telemedicine or telephone consultation in patients with acute stroke. *Curr Neurol Neurosci Rep* 2011; **11**: 42–51.
2. Demaerschalk BM. Telestrokologists: treating stroke patients here, there, and everywhere with telemedicine. *Semin Neurol* 2010; **30**: 477–91.
3. Schwamm LH, Holloway RG, Amarenco P, et al. A review of the evidence for the use of telemedicine within stroke systems of care. A scientific statement from the American Heart Association/ American Stroke Association. *Stroke* 2009; **40**: 2616–34.

4. Adeoye O, Hornung R, Khatri P, Kleindorfer D. Recombinant tissue-type plasminogen activator use for ischemic stroke in the United States: a doubling of treatment rates over the course of 5 years. *Stroke* 2011; **42**: 1952–5.

5. Miley ML, Demaerschalk BM, Olmstead NL, et al. The state of emergency stroke resources and care in rural Arizona: a platform for telemedicine. *Telemed J E Health* 2009; **15**: 691–9.

6. Demaerschalk BM. Seamless integrated stroke telemedicine systems of care: a potential solution for acute stroke care delivery delays and inefficiencies. *Stroke* 2011; **42**: 1507–8.

7. Gonzalez MA, Hanna N, Rodrigo ME, et al. Reliability of prehospital real-time cellular video phone in assessing the simplified National Institutes of Health Stroke Scale in patients with acute stroke, a novel telemedicine technology. *Stroke* 2011; **42**: 1522–7.

8. Anderson ER, Smith B, Ido M, Frankel M. Remote assessment of stroke using the iPhone 4. *J Stroke Cerebrovasc Dis*, in press.

9. Takao H, Murayama Y, Ishibashi T, et al. A new support system using a mobile device (smartphone) for diagnostic image display and treatment of stroke. *Stroke* 2012; **43**: 236–9.

10. Schwamm LH, Audebert HJ, Amarenco P, et al. Recommendations for the implementation of telemedicine within stroke systems of care. A policy statement from the American Heart Association/American Stroke Association. *Stroke* 2009; **40**: 2635–60.

11. Miley ML, Demaerschalk BM, Olmstead NL, et al. The state of emergency stroke resources and care in rural Arizona: a platform for telemedicine. *Telemed J E Health* 2009; **15**: 691–9.

12. Demaerschalk BM, Bobrow BJ, Raman R, et al., STRokE DOC AZ TIME Investigators. Stroke team remote evaluation using a digital observation camera in Arizona: the initial Mayo clinic experience trial. *Stroke* 2010; **41**: 1251–8.

13. Linkous JD. Telestroke and telemedicine: national trends, reimbursement, and what's ahead. American Telemedicine Association. www.americantelemed.org.

14. Demaerschalk BM, Hwang HM, Leung G. Cost analysis review of stroke centers, telestroke, and rt-PA. *Am J Manag Care* 2010; **16**: 537–44.

15. Nelson RE, Saltzman GM, Skalabrin EJ, et al. The cost-effectiveness of telestroke in the treatment of acute ischemic stroke. *Neurology* 2011; **77**: 1590–8.

16. Switzer JA, Demaerschalk BM, Xie J, et al. Cost-effectiveness of hub-and-spoke telestroke networks for the management of acute ischemic stroke from the hospitals' perspective. *Circ Cardiovasc Qual Outcomes* 2012, in press. (Abstract.)

17. Liu CF. Key factors influencing the intention of telecare adoption: an institutional perspective. *Telemed J E Health* 2011; **17**: 288–93.

18. Silva GS, Viswanathan A, Shandra E, Schwamm LH. Telestroke 2010: a survey of currently active stroke telemedicine programs in the US. *Stroke* 2011; **42**: e292 (Abstract).

19. Rogove HJ, McArthur D, Demaerschalk BM, Vespa PM. Barriers to telemedicine: survey of current users in acute care units. *Telemed J E Health* 2012; **18**: 1–6.

20. Hess DC, Switzer JA. Stroke telepresence, Removing all geographic barriers. *Neurology* 2011; **76**: 1121–3.

21. Martin-Schild S, Morales MM, Khaja AM, et al. Is the drip-and-ship approach to delivering thrombolysis for acute ischemic stroke safe? *J Emerg Med* 2011; **41**: 135–141.

9

Appendix: Practical Clinical Stroke Scales

Kevin M. Barrett, MD, MSc and James F. Meschia, MD

Department of Neurology, Mayo Clinic Florida, Jacksonville, Florida

Introduction

The purpose of this appendix is to provide the reader with validated and commonly utilized clinical stroke scales and their scoring paradigms in an easy-to-access format and location. Scales used to measure stroke severity, functional status, and stroke-related disability are included. Clinical severity scores commonly used after hemorrhagic stroke are provided. A clinical scale for risk stratification after atrial fibrillation is provided. Eligibility criteria for intravenous rt-PA from 0–3 hours and 3–4.5 hours are summarized. Finally, an internet link to a complete listing of acute stroke clinical trials with status updates is included.

Stroke clinical outcome scales

Table 9.1 Modified Rankin score

Score	Definition
0	No symptoms
1	No significant disability. Able to carry out all usual activities, despite some symptoms.
2	Slight disability. Able to look after own affairs without assistance, but unable to carry out all previous activities.
3	Moderate disability. Requires some help, but able to walk unassisted.
4	Moderately severe disability. Unable to attend to own bodily needs without assistance, and unable to walk unassisted.
5	Severe disability. Requires constant nursing care and attention, bedridden, incontinent.
6	Death

A Modified Rankin Score of 0 or 1 at 3 months post rt-PA or placebo treatment was considered to be favorable outcome in the NINDS and the ECASS III studies. In the PROACT II study, an MRS of ≤2 was considered to be favorable outcome.

Stroke, First Edition. Edited by Kevin M. Barrett and James F. Meschia.
© 2013 John Wiley & Sons, Ltd. Published 2013 by John Wiley & Sons, Ltd.

Table 9.2 Barthel index

Instructions: Record information about function for the 24 hours before the assessment. Take the information from the best available source (for example, nurses, relatives, the patient). Comatose patients are given a score of "0" even if they have not yet been incontinent of feces.

Feeding	☐	0 = dependent
	☐	5 = needs help e.g. cutting, spreading butter
	☐	10 = independent in all actions
Bowels	☐	0 = incontinent
	☐	5 = occasional accident
	☐	10 = continent
Bladder	☐	0 = incontinent/catheterized and unable to manage
	☐	5 = occasional accident
	☐	10 = continent
Grooming	☐	0 = needs help
	☐	5 = independent for face/hair/teeth/shaving
Toilet use	☐	0 = dependent
	☐	5 = needs some help
	☐	10 = independent
Transfers (bed-chair)	☐	0 = unable with transfers
	☐	5 = major help with transfers, but sits without support
	☐	10 = minor help (verbal or physical)
	☐	15 = independent
Walking	☐	0 = unable
	☐	5 = independent in wheelchair
	☐	10 = walks with help of person (verbal or physical)
	☐	15 = independent (may use aid)
Dressing	☐	0 = dependent
	☐	5 = needs help, but does half
	☐	10 = independent (including buttons/zips/laces)
Stairs	☐	0 = unable
	☐	5 = needs help (verbal or physical)
	☐	10 = independent
Bathing	☐	0 = dependent
	☐	5 = independent

Table 9.3 National Institutes of Health Stroke Scale[a]

Category	Scale definition
1a. Level of consciousness	0=Alert 1=Not alert, arousable 2=Not alert, obtunded 3=Unresponsive
1b. Questions	0=Answers both correctly 1=Answers one correctly 2=Answers neither correctly
1c. Commands	0=Performs both tasks correctly 1=Performs one task correctly 2=Performs neither task
2. Gaze	0=Normal 1=Partial gaze palsy 2=Total gaze palsy
3. Visual fields	0=No visual loss 1=Partial hemianopsia 2=Complete hemianopsia 3=Bilateral hemianopsia
4. Facial palsy	0=Normal 1=Minor paralysis 2=Partial paralysis 3=Complete paralysis
5a. Left motor arm	0=No drift 1=Drift before 10 s 2=Falls before 10 s 3=No effort against gravity 4=No movement
5b. Right motor arm	0=No drift 1=Drift before 10 s 2=Falls before 10 s 3=No effort against gravity 4=No movement
6a. Left motor leg	0=No drift 1=Drift before 5 s 2=Falls before 5 s 3=No effort against gravity 4=No movement
6b. Right motor leg	0=No drift 1=Drift before 5 s 2=Falls before 5 s 3=No effort against gravity 4=No movement
7. Ataxia	0=Absent 1=One limb 2=Two limbs
8. Sensory	0=Normal 1=Mild loss 2=Severe loss

(*Continued*)

Table 9.3 (*cont'd*)

Category	Scale definition
9. Language	0=Normal 1=Mild aphasia 2=Severe aphasia 3=Mute or global aphasia
10. Dysarthria	0=Normal 1=Mild 2=Severe
11. Extinction/inattention	0=Normal 1=Mild 2=Severe

[a] The full NIHSS with instructions and scoring sheet is available online at http://www.ninds.nih.gov/doctors/NIH_Stroke_Scale.pdf.
Reprinted with permission from Adams HP Jr, del Zoppo G, Alberts MJ, et al. Guidelines for the early management of adults with ischemic stroke: a guideline from the American Heart Association/American Stroke Council, Clinical Cardiology Council, Cardiovascular Radiology and Intervention Council, and the Atherosclerotic Peripheral Vascular Disease and Quality of Care Outcomes in Research Interdisciplinary Working Groups: the American Academy of Neurology affirms the value of this guideline as an educational tool for neurologists [published errata appears in *Stroke* 2007; **38**(6): e38 and *Stroke* 2007; **38**(9): e96]. *Stroke* 2007; **38**(6): 1655–711.

Clinical risk stratification scores

Table 9.4 CHADS2 score for persistent or paroxysmal nonvalvular atrial fibrillation

CHADS2 score
Congestive heart failure history (1 point)
Hypertension history (1 point)
Age ≥75 (1 point)
Diabetes mellitus history (1 point)
Stroke symptoms or TIA (2 points)

Score	Annual stroke risk (%)
0	1.9
1	2.8
2	4.0
3	5.9
4	8.5
5	12.5
6	18.2

Table 9.5 CTA "spot sign" score for predicting risk of hematoma expansion

Spot sign finding	Points
Number of spot signs	
1–2	1
≥3	2
Maximal axial length	
1–4 mm	0
≥5 mm	1
Maximum density (in Hounsfield Units, HU)	
120–179 HU	0
180 HU	1

Spot sign score	Risk of bleed growth (%)
0	2
1	33
2	50
3	94
4	100

The "spot sign" score is the sum of the individual components listed above; when multiple "spots" are present, the maximal measurements are obtained from the largest one. Note also that the recommended HU cut-off values for density are based on the specific CTA acquisition protocol used in the paper by Delgado Almandoz et al. (Delgado Almandoz JE, Yoo AJ, Stone MJ, et al. The spot sign score in primary intracerebral hemorrhage identifies patients at highest risk of in-hospital mortality and poor outcome among survivors. *Stroke* 2010; **41**: 54–60), and may not be generalizable to other CTA protocols using different contrast agents, injection rates, and timing of imaging.

Hemorrhagic stroke severity scales

Table 9.6 Hunt and Hess and World Federation of Neurological Surgeons score for subarachnoid hemorrhage

	Hunt–Hess	WFNS
I	Asymptomatic or mild headache	GCS score 15 without hemiparesis
II	Moderate to severe headache, nuchal rigidity, no focal deficits other than cranial nerve palsy	GCS score 13–14 without hemiparesis
III	Confusion, lethargy, or mild focal deficits other than cranial nerve palsy	GCS score 13–14 with hemiparesis
IV	Stupor or moderate to severe hemiparesis	GCS score 7–12
V	Coma, extensor posturing, moribund appearance	GCS score 3–6

GCS, Glasgow Coma Scale; WFNS, World Federation of Neurological Surgeons score.

Table 9.7 Radiographic scales used to grade patients with subarachnoid hemorrhage

	Fisher scale	Modified Fisher scale
0		No SAH or IVH
1	No SAH or IVH	Minimum* or thin SAH, no IVH
2	Diffuse, thin SAH, no clot >1 mm in thickness	Minimum or thin SAH, with IVH
3	Localized thick subarachnoid clot >1 mm in thickness	Thick SAH, no IVH
4	Predominant IVH or intracerebral hemorrhage without thick SAH	Thick SAH, with IVH

*The definition of "thick" is at least 5 mm.
IVH, intraventricular hemorrhage; SAH, subarachnoid hemorrhage.

Eligibility criteria for intravenous rt-PA 0–4.5 hours

Table 9.8 Exclusion criteria for intravenous rt-PA <3 hours after symptom onset

CT or MRI evidence of intracranial hemorrhage
Rapidly resolving or minor and isolated deficit
Caution in severely affected, obtunded or comatose patients
Seizure with postictal deficits
Symptoms suggestive of subarachnoid hemorrhage
History of previous intracranial hemorrhage
Head trauma or prior stroke in previous 3 months
Myocardial infarction in previous 3 months
Gastrointestinal or urinary tract hemorrhage in previous 21 days
Major surgery in previous 14 days
Arterial puncture at a noncompressible site in previous 7 days
Blood pressure persistently elevated >185 mmHg systolic and >105 mmHg diastolic
Active bleeding or acute trauma (fracture) on examination
International Normalized Ratio (INR) >1.7
Prolonged aPTT if heparin received in previous 48 hours
Platelet count ≤100,000/µL
Blood glucose ≤50 mg/dL
CT evidence of multilobar infarction (hypodensity >1/3 cerebral hemisphere)

Table 9.9 Exclusion criteria for intravenous rt-PA 3–4.5 hours

Same as 0–3 hours exclusion criteria AND:
    Age >80 years
    On oral anticoagulation (independent of INR)
    Baseline NIH Stroke Scale score >25
    A history of stroke AND diabetes

Internet resources

A complete listing of acute stroke clinical trials with status updates can be found at http://www.stroke center.org/trials/clinicalstudies/list.

Index

Note: Page numbers in *italics* refer to Figures; those in **bold** to Tables.

Stroke, First Edition. Edited by Kevin M. Barrett and James F. Meschia.
© 2013 John Wiley & Sons, Ltd. Published 2013 by John Wiley & Sons, Ltd.